THE MODERN METHOD
OF BIRTH CONTROL

The Modern Method

OF

Birth Control

By

THURSTON SCOTT WELTON, M.D., F.A.C.S.

Editor of *The American Journal of Surgery*

Emeritus Clinical Professor of
Obstetrics and Gynecology,
State University
of New York, College
of Medicine.

GROSSET & DUNLAP
Publishers   New York

*"Nature is not to be governed
except through obeying her."*

—Francis Bacon, Lord Verulam

TABLE OF CONTENTS

TABLE OF CONTENTS

PREFACE

Twenty years ago few women knew about and followed The Modern or "rhythmic" Method of Birth Control. But for years scientific observers have been trying to fix the exact time of fertile and sterile menstrual cycles. About 1925, two internationally famed scientists, working unknown to each other, reached the same conclusion as to when "safe" and "unsafe" periods occur. Well known scientists confirmed their findings with studies of married couples who had used the "method" over a long period of time. Not one pregnancy was reported by any couple who followed the system faithfully. Following these early reports, articles began to appear in the American literature on the subject and during the past two decades the Modern Method has been recommended by thousands of physicians.

Although most people practice the Modern Method to avoid conception, it is interesting to observe that a large number of physicians use it for treating cases of sterility. When physicians ask The Journal of the American Medical Association how to treat sterility in the female, the invariable answer, among other suggestions, is that intercourse *must* occur during the "fertile period" in the menstrual cycle and not during the "sterile period."

The Modern or Rhythmic Method of Birth Control

shows you how to determine when fertility and sterility occur every month—in other words, when intercourse is "safe" and when it is "unsafe."

You will be told, as we have been told many times, that the method is not "safe." Usually, unconvinced physicians say that they know or have heard of one or two cases in which it failed. Whenever such reported cases are investigated, it is found that the method is not at fault but the way the method is followed. At times the method should not be put into practice.

On the other hand, out of the hundreds of letters telling us how perfectly the method has proved itself, there have been only a few letters of complaint. Among our medical friends are many who prescribe the "method" in their daily practice. They report that from what they have observed, they have no reason to date to change this prescription.

The vast majority of women who have adopted this method of avoiding pregnancy are members of the Catholic Church. It is not contrary to the teaching of this church because the Modern Method teaches AVOIDANCE and not CONTRACEPTION. It works with nature and not against nature.

It is not unreasonable to assume that if the thousands of Catholic women who have relied solely on this system found it unsafe, they would have made mass protests to their physicians. In turn, these physicians would have written articles for medical journals telling the profession that the "method" was something fit for the medical junk pile. Finally, Catholic clergymen could not and would not continue to suggest the "method" to their following, if they believed it was unreliable.

Under the headline, "Marital Forum Conducted for Catholic Youth" in the New York Herald Tribune (April 4, 1938), I chanced to read the following: "A girl asked whether rhythmic cycles (The Modern Method) were considered reliable in the average woman. The physician answered in the affirmative and added it was unreliable in less than 10 per cent." Learning from their Catholic friends and acquaintances that this system is safe and reliable, many women of other religious beliefs have put their stamp of approval on the Modern Method of Birth Control.

We close with this advice. In order to practice the Modern Method successfully, it is most essential for a woman to know her particular menstrual cycle. This knowledge must be based on facts and not on guess work. Physicians' studies of thousands of mature women reveal that very few women have regular menstrual cycles and that most healthy women have a variation of from one to four days over a period of many months. A woman should write down the dates of her menstrual periods, for only in this way can she really know in what particular cycle she fits.

The chance of failure is slight, provided the woman truly knows the actual variation of her menstrual cycle and faithfully follows the useful charts which appear in the back of this volume.

THURSTON SCOTT WELTON

THE MODERN METHOD
OF BIRTH CONTROL

CHAPTER I

Biologically speaking, the fundamental purpose of love is the continuity of the race. Human beings, especially in civilized countries, marry and—as a result of this civil and religious ceremony, permitting the union of the sexes—the earth is populated. Among civilized peoples marriage is the stamp of social approval.

Love and marriage are intimately connected. Both are the subjects of day-dreams and fiction; we find them expressed in poetry, and in the manners, morals and institutions of every community.

Scientifically viewed, marriage is more than the successful ending of a courtship. It has been said that love and the institution of marriage are but the tricks of Nature aiming at the endless reproduction of human beings. For love leads to sexual intimacy, and this in turn leads to the procreation of children. In addition, marriage imposes duties of economic coöperation. Usually it is celebrated in a public and solemn manner, after receiving, as a sacrament, the blessings of religion. We are told that in primitive and civilized countries alike marriage, as a sacrament, is protected by spiritual powers. The religious aspect of marriage is closely related to the legal, in that it adds to "the validity and

3

sanctity of other functions, rather than establishing new ones."

Marriage is not limited to mere cohabitation. In no society are those of the opposite sex permitted to share a life in common and produce children without the approval of the community and according to its religious and civil laws. We quote from the *Encyclopædia Britannica:*

"Marriage is the most important legal contract in every human society, the one which refers to the continuity of the race; it implies a most delicate and difficult adjustment of a passionate and emotional relationship with domestic coöperation; it involves the cohabitation of male and female, perennially attracted and yet in many ways forever incompatible; it focuses in a difficult personal relationship of two people of the interest of wider groups; of the progeny, of their parents, of their kindred, and in fact of the whole community."

Summed up in a few words, among civilized people marriage is for the purpose of creating a home and bearing children.

From ancient times man has attempted in various ways to prevent conception. For one reason or another he has desired to prevent or limit offspring. He is an animal that cohabits at all times, the act not being restricted to certain periods, as it is among many of the other animals. Therefore, the marriage act is more than likely to occasion the pregnant state. Owing to any of several factors—lust, selfishness, economic reasons, too many children born in rapid succession, poor health or serious disease in the parents (especially the woman), the desire for freedom from parental care and responsibility—the need for birth control has come, especially in recent times, into the conscious minds of a large proportion of the population.

In many states of our own country as well as in many foreign countries the dissemination of birth-control knowledge as well as its practice has been illegal. The Catholic Church and certain other religious bodies have never sanctioned the use of contraceptives. Their thesis has been that the union of the sexes is a God-given function intended for creating in the likeness of the parents, and that any chemical or mechanical contrivance intended for thwarting this purpose is contrary to the laws of Nature and of the Church.

Every physician knows there has been no method devised or recommended with the prevention of conception as its object that is 100 per cent perfect or certain in its efficacy. In addition, many methods devised for birth-control are repulsive except to the hardened and calloused. To the women of refinement, possessed of noble sensibilities, they are unæsthetic and revolting. Certain mechanical contrivances have led to serious illness, chronic invalidism or death. The proponents of artificial methods of preventing conception, in their detailed statistical reports, show that their methods are about 93 per cent effective. Until the Cycle of Safety—Nature's method—was discovered, there has been no ideal method, although man has been experimenting for years in the hope of discovering a satisfactory something by which he might control the time of impregnation. We recite these facts to impress the reader with the futility of such chemical and mechanical means, some potent for danger, and to offer the assurance that the method which will be explained gives as good end-results, if not better, is free from any danger, is in truth Nature's own method, and has the approval of religious bodies.

The attitude of the Catholic Church was summed up by His Eminence, Cardinal Bourne, Archbishop of Westminster, who said, "There is no law requiring married people to have large families, and if they wish to live in continence they are entitled to do so, but they are absolutely forbidden to exercise the act of generation *and frustrate* its natural purpose."

This means that it is no sin to refrain from intercourse at any time; the individual may exercise his own judgment and wish as to when he cohabits. But should he cohabit he may not, by any artificial means or by any perversion, try to prevent the biological consequences of that act. In other words, neither the man nor the woman may in any way try to prevent conception as a result of their union.

Nature's method of control calls for normal intercourse. It is entirely divorced from any unnatural manner of union; there is no employment of any chemical or gadget in association with it. It calls for normal relations, but also calls for continence during a certain period in the menstrual cycle if children are not desired. As we shall learn there is a time in the menstrual cycle of women in which continence must be practiced. At all other times normal intercourse is permitted. Inasmuch as this is according to Nature the Church gives it its approval.

It is a blessing to mankind that this method has been discovered, since there are times when even the most loving, moral, and religious people have a sincere desire and good reason to limit or prevent, for the time being, the bringing of children, or additional children into the world. Physicians know that in some cases that the bearing of too many children in rapid succession is not good for the health of the mother. Often a woman is found to be afflicted with an illness that might make her an invalid were she to become pregnant. There are diseases that are likely to cause death should they complicate pregnancy or should pregnancy complicate them. Economic factors often make it desirable to stop, at least for the time being, the bearing of children. For reasons peculiar to themselves some parents wish to space their offspring, bringing their babies into the world at designated intervals of time.

But because there has been no scientific, reliable method which legally and religiously permitted them to follow such preferences, married people often resorted to unnatural means that reacted unfavorably on their health and mental happiness. These objections are now no longer in order. Husband and wife may have natural relations at certain times of the month without the apprehensive fear of a pregnancy not desired at that time. They can learn at what times they are to abstain from marital relations, unless they desire a baby. No longer need wives send their husbands to a drug store to procure a special jelly, a suppository, powder or other contrivance, all uncertain in their action and likely to fail in the end—for they will fail, at best, seven times out of every hundred. No longer need the harassed woman seek a birth-control clinic or a physician's office, often at great cost, to seek information concerning the *modus operandi* of adjusting a mechanical contrivance, or else to have adjusted into her cervix (neck of the womb) some rubber, metal or glass affair—some device which has a history of countless failures, and which any gynecologist will tell you has caused pelvic infection, has been the etiological factor leading to a pelvic condition often necessitating an abdominal operation, and which in many cases has made women sterile or invalids, and in others has been the cause of death. In time, when women are educated in this simple, natural method, calling for the expenditure of no money, but demanding only that they exercise intelligent care as to the time of the month they cohabit, a prolific source of the troubles peculiar to women will be eliminated.

From reports of physicians throughout the country who are advising their patients to practise Nature's method of control it is noticed that so imbedded in the lay-minds is the use of chemical and mechanical means to prevent conception, that women hesitate to accept heart and soul this simple method.

Man, in the laboratory and in the clinic, has merely discovered a method which Nature has been offering him since the dawn of time. In a later chapter we shall learn how these discoveries were made. We shall learn how they have been tested clinically. Meanwhile a few authentic statistics are offered: A. G. Miller reported (*Surgery, Gynecology and Obstetrics,* the official journal of the American College of Surgeons) sexual union 354 times during the post-menstrual sterility time, and 371 times in the period during the pre-menstrual sterility time (725 times in all), and in *NO CASE DID PREGNANCY OCCUR;* Schroeder had no discordant results in 100 observed cases; Rugell, had 2 discordant results in 106 cases; while Wintz, out of 27 observed cases, had no discordant cases. All of these are physicians whose findings and reports are accepted without question by the medical profession.

Both Ogino and Knaus, who are credited with discovering this method, report uniformly excellent results. *From available statistics the method is reliable in 97 per cent of all cases.*

Physicians have used controlled cases in which the women have reported at frequent intervals of time, and full data concerning their menstrual cycles, symptoms and dates of marital union have been charted for study. The conclusions drawn were that during the sterile times of the menstrual period cohabitation would not be followed by pregnancy. In those controlled cases in which the patient desired to become pregnant, intercourse took place during the fertile period of the menstrual cycle with happy results.

The *Modern Method* is like a two-bladed sword—it cuts both ways. It offers a time for the exercise of nuptial rights during which it is well-nigh impossible for the wife to become pregnant. On the other hand, for those desiring pregnancy, it indicates the best time to cohabit in order to attain this end. Workers in this field of medicine have advised women of their sterile times, and these women did not become pregnant until they desired children, at which time they cohabited during the fertile periods, and became with child. The *Modern Method* is simply one of *knowing when to abstain* from intercourse if one *does not wish to become pregnant,* or of *knowing when to cohabit* if *pregnancy is wished.*

The *Modern Method is not birth-control* in the accepted sense of the term. Birth-control, as popularly understood, is artificial contraception, whereas this method is natural control. It asks the woman to purchase nothing. No mechanical or medicated contrivance is required. *Husband and wife have natural intercourse.* The *Modern Method* demands but one sacrifice, if it can be called that, namely: *Intercourse must be restricted to certain fixed times. Marital relations at definite, known times in the menstrual cycle is the whole story of the natural method.* If relations are restricted to these times, according to reliable figures, the margin of error is about 3 per cent. Because these statistics are equal to—if not slightly better than—those reported by the better-known advocates of birth-control, when women become aware of these facts this natural method will doubtless be the method of choice.

Because the *Modern Method* simply means control of the will as to when intercourse may be indulged in, and is in no way a method of prevention, it is sanctioned by the Catholic Church, as well as by other religious bodies.

How and why the *Modern Method* is based on scientifically proved facts will be explained in the following chapters.

CHAPTER II

THE EGG AND THE MALE CELL

Let us begin with the female at birth and note the changes that take place until she is a matured woman capable of bearing children.

At birth there is little differentiation between a girl and a boy. But during the early years each takes on different, marked characteristics. By the time they walk the differentiation is apparent. Sexually, a change begins in the girl about the time she reaches the age of ten years. This transformation becomes more apparent when she is from twelve to fourteen years old. At that time she reaches the age of puberty—she has become a woman. Biologically, she is capable of reproduction. This phase of her life continues until she has almost completed the fifth decade of existence, when she goes through what is called "the change of life" or menopause. At the menopause a woman ceases to be capable of reproduction. She has reached her Indian summer.

When the girl emerges into a woman there are marked physical and psychic changes that take place in her body and mind. The pelvis enlarges. It takes on the size and shape necessary for her main function in life. She becomes rounded out with fat and suddenly has a "figure." Former angles or dumpy shapelessness are now replaced by graceful curves and pleasant proportions. The breasts enlarge, the nipples become more prominent and are surrounded by a small circle of discoloration (primary areola). The skin takes on an increased activity, especially the sebaceous glands. At the beginning of puberty, because the sebaceous glands suddenly become active, skin eruptions, such as acne or blackheads (comedones) are likely to occur. The hair becomes thicker and of a fine texture. The external genitals undergo a change; they enlarge and grow darker, and the blood supply increases. The thyroid (a gland situated in the mid-section of the front of the neck) enlarges and plays an important role in her life. Her voice changes, usually becoming fuller and more melodious.

At the onset of puberty the girl's mind changes. Usually for a while she is liable to hysterical manifestations; she will cry, laugh and sing without rhyme or reason. Her will is uncertain and capricious. Once her new status is fully developed, however, and her habits fixed, these emotional storms subside and she continues her existence on a more even mental keel. About this time she begins to notice the male in a different light. As time goes on her interest in him may increase, as does her modesty. However, unless awakened by some outside, artificial means her sex urge remains quiescent and often does not fully develop until after marriage.

When she walks through the door from girlhood into womanhood other internal changes take place. A marked increase occurs in the size of the womb and other organs of generation. Her ductless glands take on new and increased functions. The egg is liberated periodically. The girl, now a woman, can become pregnant. But although she is capable of reproduction, at this time she is totally unfit to bring forth children. There have been reported cases of motherhood at incredibly early ages, but such young women are to be pitied. The pelvis does not reach its full growth until the eighteenth to twentieth year. Authorities who have studied this problem tell us that in those living in the temperate zone pregnancy had best be deferred until the female is from twenty to twenty-two years old.

Every so often an egg is liberated from an ovary. When this occurs for the first time usually it is followed by the first menstruation. As we shall learn, menstruation is the result of an egg not being fertilized. Therefore, menstruation, the most prominent sign of maturity, is dependent on ovulation, though we know now that in some cases this is not always true. This is a rare phenomena. Its importance is mainly concerned with cases of sterility. Pregnancy, sterility, ovulation and menstruation are bound with one string, and to understand the cycle of the safe and unsafe periods we must have some knowledge of these phenomena.

Before we can thoroughly understand them, however, we must know something concerning the anatomy peculiar to the female. A great many women go through life knowing little or nothing about themselves; or, at best, their conceptions of how they are made are fantastic.

The vagina, which may be likened to a tube, is the depository of the father-cells as a result of physical union. At its upper end is the womb. The virgin womb is shaped like a flattened pear. Roughly, it is about the size of an average pear. It has a cavity which opens into the vagina. At the sides of the womb, near its top, are the openings of the two Fallopian tubes, one tube on each side. Each tube leads to an ovary attached by a ligament to the outside of the womb and at its rear.

The womb in health is movable, and is held in place by certain supports and ligaments. Usually it makes almost a right angle to the vagina, with its fundus (top) directed toward the front of the body. It is behind and below the symphysis pubis (the bony structure felt in the front of the lowest, middle portion of the abdomen). The womb is a muscular organ and has been called "the heart of the pelvis" because it contracts and retracts at times. The cavity of the womb has a glandular lining that plays a major part in menstruation and pregnancy. This lining is called the endometrium.

The womb is a special organ. Nature has given it to woman for just one purpose—the reception of the fertilized egg and its implantation, and for harboring and safeguarding the products of conception until a full-term baby emerges into the world. If women laid their eggs as fishes or hens do. Nature would not have given them wombs. Except for the purpose of pregnancy a womb is a useless organ. Just as we have teeth with which to chew food, and bones in order that we may walk, so a woman has a womb that she may bear babies.

The Fallopian tube is about as long as your finger. There are two of them, one running out from each side of the uterus. Their diameter is about that of the straw that one uses for his drink. The inner end terminates in the cavity of the womb; the outer end is free, close to the ovary, and is slightly trumpet-shaped and finger-like. The egg gets into the outer end of the tube and passes through. It is during its journey through the tube that it is met by the father-cells, one of which fertilizes it.

The ovaries are the main organs responsible for the sex characteristics of the female. As we have learned, when a girl reaches the age of twelve to fourteen years she undergoes a marked physical and mental change and becomes a woman. These changes are the result of activities and changes in the ovaries. The ovaries throw hormones (an inner secretion) into the bloodstream, and these internal secretions, in conjunction with the hormones of other ductless glands, play a paramount part in her body structure, her mental outlook, and her happiness and usefulness in life.

Should the ovaries be removed or their function ended by disease, radium or X-Rays, the woman goes through an artificial change of life, menstruation ceases and pregnancy becomes impossible.

Therefore, the ovaries have a twofold function: To form and liberate ova (eggs), and to produce hormones that are essential to health.

We now have reached an important part of our study: the manufacture and freeing of the female cell or egg.

In the child the greater portion of the ovary is filled with large numbers of undeveloped eggs. Those nearest the central part of the ovary show the most advanced stages of development. In young women the ovary still contains large numbers of these undeveloped eggs. Each egg has a nucleus (the comparatively large body within and usually near the center of any typical cell). Occasionally, an undeveloped egg may contain more than one nucleus.

The egg becomes larger. From birth until the change of life, closed sacs which contain the egg (Graafian follicles) are constantly being developed. Before the girl reaches puberty they are found only in the deeper parts of the ovary and do not reach the surface. Later on, however, these follicles containing the egg make their way to the surface and become transparent. As a follicle approaches the surface of the ovary its walls become thinner. The egg becomes much larger as it approaches maturity. As the Graafian follicle reaches its fullest maturity it ruptures, and the egg is extruded and finds its way into a tube.

The freeing of the egg from its follicle is called *ovulation*. When the first egg is liberated it is usually followed in about a couple of weeks by menstruation, provided the egg remains sterile. With the beginning of ovulation and menstruation the girl is transformed into a woman.

In the vast majority of women one egg is freed in each menstrual cycle. From the depths of the ovary the egg moves towards the surface and develops, the follicle bursts and the egg is liberated. And this process is continuous during the childbearing life of the woman. If ovulation is constant and regular, then menstruation, as a rule, is constant and regular. If some irregular condition interferes with ovulation, then the menstrual cycle becomes variable and pathological.

To understand and have confidence in the theory of fixed cycles of sterility and fertility (the times when pregnancy is and is not possible) it is necessary to remember that it has been discovered that ovulation (freeing of the egg) occurs from 12 to 16 days *before* the advent of menstruation. In other words—and this is hard for many laymen to comprehend—a woman menstruates, and *12 to 16 days before the next menstruation is due to occur the egg is freed*. If it is fertilized, that next menstruation does not occur because the woman is pregnant. If the egg does not become fertilized by the father-cell, then—12 to 16 days after ovulation—menstruation takes place.

This point of *time* in the menstrual cycle of ovulation

is one of the foundations upon which has been built the theory of the safe and unsafe periods in the matter of pregnancy.

For years hundreds of scientific investigators have been attempting to fix the exact time of ovulation in the human menstrual cycle. Then, two scientists, of international reputation, working independently and unknown to each other at the time, arrived at almost the same conclusions. Professor K. Ogino of Niigata, Japan, determined that ovulation occurs 12 to 16 days prior to the next expected menstruation; while Dr. Herman Knaus, of the University Women's Clinic in Graz, Austria, placed the ovulation time at 14 to 16 days prior to the expected period. Other well known scientists have concurred in these findings (for the difference between Ogino's and Knaus' findings is unimportant). Some of these scientists are Dr. Allen, Dr. Hartman, Professor Fraenkel of Breslau, Professor Schroeder of Kiel, and Dr. Shaw of England. This by no means exhausts the list of the prominent workers who agree with Ogino and Knaus—their names would make a long list.

How did Ogino and Knaus make their discoveries? Dr. Ogino, being one of the foremost gynecologists of Japan, had an opportunity of studying the ovaries of many women upon whom he did abdominal operations. From his intensive study of the ovaries, of the stage of development of the follicle, and of the "yellow body" (about which we shall learn shortly), he noted their relation to the ensuing menstruation. As a result of these observations he concluded that ovulation occurs 12 to 16 days before the next menstruation. This method has been followed by other investigators with the same results. Ogino recorded that ovulation took place 12 to 16 days before the menses in all but fifteen cases in 557 women. These fifteen women did not fit the pattern, owing either to pelvic diseases which affect ovulation or to his inability to get accurate case-histories.

Dr. Knaus approached the problem from a different angle—from the viewpoint of endocrinology (the science of the internal secretions).

The posterior lobe of the pituitary gland (situated at the base of the brain) manufactures a secretion which is thrown into the blood-stream. This hormone or internal secretion stimulates the muscular contractions of the uterus.

After the egg has been freed it leaves a cavity in the ovary which becomes filled with blood. In turn, this blood-clot is absorbed. By an unknown process the space which was occupied by this blood-clot becomes filled with cells having yellow color. These constitute the *corpus luteum,* or "yellow body."

Let us imagine that this corpus luteum (or yellow body) is aware that an egg has been sent out on its journey in the hope that it will meet a male companion (a father-cell) and, so become fertilized; and knowing that, should fertilization occur, the egg's destination is the cavity of the womb, this corpus luteum by way of the blood-stream then sends out an internal secretion with a message to the womb commanding it to make ready to receive an important tenant. Another message goes to the muscles of the womb telling them to eliminate the action of the hormone of the pituitary gland, which, as we have stated, causes the contraction and retraction of the womb muscles. The muscles obey this message, contractions cease and the womb becomes prepared to house the fertilized egg.

With these facts to work from, Dr. Knaus knew that if he could discover when this yellow body begins to function he could then determine when ovulation takes place. He accordingly injected a small quantity of pituitrin into a woman's blood-stream. With a special instrument (a manometer) he noted the effect on the womb. If, as a result of the injection, the womb contracted and expanded, he knew that the yellow body had not begun to function. But if the yellow body had begun to function, he knew that the uterus would remain inactive following the injection, and that ovulation had taken place. He repeated this experiment numberless times, and as a result of them he placed the time of ovulation 14 to 16 days prior to menstruation. After he published his findings his work was checked by scientists in all parts of the world.

In *Colorado Medicine* (June, 1933), Dr. Cyrus W. Anderson wrote an article concerning his observations, which were to the effect that women become conscious of a peculiar sensation in the pelvis at about the middle of the menstrual cycle. Dr. Anderson describes this sensation as "mild, cramp-like pain coming on suddenly, followed by a sort of bearing-down sensation or feeling as if the bottom had dropped out of the pelvis, and lasting a couple of hours. . . . It is unlike any other sort of pain." He concluded that the pain was caused by the rupture of the ovary in the freeing of an ovum. He states that, reasoning from the time of this intermenstrual pain, he placed the sterile period, for those of his patients who wished to space their births, at four days after the time of pain. ". . . And not in a single case has there been a pregnancy in patients using this safe period," he recorded. However, this symptom of "middle-pain" is not given much weight, by a majority of workers, as associated with ovulation.

Dr. Wilfred Shaw, writing in the *British Medical Journal* (January 6, 1934) on "Ovulation and Menstruation," studied the ovaries in thirty-six cases in which women with a twenty-eight day cycle underwent operations for various causes. In addition, he collected forty-nine cases in which the womb alone was removed. In twenty-one of the patients in whom the ovaries were examined the uterus was studied histologically. In practically all of the cases so examined for the presence of a ruptured follicle or corpus luteum the evidence was clear that ovulation occurs about the fourteenth day of the menstrual cycle. There has been a belief among embryologists that ovulation can be provoked by intercourse. Apparently most authorities are unwilling to accept this belief so far as it relates to the human being, although conceding its possibilities in animals in a lower scale.

And so today, among a great many physicians, it is an accepted fact that the egg is freed from the ovary and starts its journey down the tube at some time from 12 to 16 days before a menstruation. If one truly believes this scientific fact then he is ready to consider other facts. If he does not believe this fact then he need no longer consider the theory of the safe and unsafe periods in the menstrual cycle. For the time of ovulation is the foundation of this theory.

If the egg lived from the time of its birth until it was cast off with the menstrual debris, there would be no so-called safe period in a woman's existence. If the egg had a long life it would be possible for a father-cell to impregnate or fertilize it at any time it was in the body. Were this true, all women living normal married lives would be in an almost constant state of pregnancy. There would be no sterile or safe time. But we do know that as a general rule one egg is expelled each month and that *it lives but a few hours* unless it is fertilized by the father-cell. Ogino wrote: "The long-life theory of an ovum is gradually coming to be challenged by recent authors, and there are therefore now few men who believe in such a theory." The duration of the fertilizable capacity time of an ovum is 12 to 24 hours after ovulation.

Now we have two scientific facts: 1. That the egg is expelled from 12 to 16 days prior to menstruation; 2. That the ovum cannot be fertilized after it is 24 hours old.

What about the father-cells?

A father-cell is called a spermatozoön. Spermatozoa are manufactured in unbelievable numbers in the male testicles. The testicles of the male are analogous to the ovaries of the female. They produce the cells necessary for reproduction. Each throws into the blood-stream hormones that make for the full development of sex and its characteristics. A spermatozoön has a spear-shaped head, and a tail. It is capable of motion. It moves by wriggling its tail. Deposited in the vagina or vulva it gains entrance to the womb, travels along the cavity of the womb, and so into the tubes. With its 200-odd million brothers (deposited at each marriage-union) it eagerly hunts for the virgin ovum. If a spermatozoön in a tube meets an ovum, it pierces it. At that moment the ovum is fertilized and the woman is pregnant. However, suppose no ovum is present in a tube. The spermatozoa then seeks in vain. Do the father-cells then wait for another ovum to appear? They do not. Have they long lives? No. It has been estimated that the father-cells lose their power of fecundation within 24 to 48 hours after entering the female organs. Dr. Knaus says: "The latest researches have brought a decided enlightenment about the life of spermatozoa. The spermatozoa lose their ability to fecundate much earlier than they stop their squirming movements. This means that their ability to move is in no way a sign of their ability to fecundate." Stuttgart also came to similar conclusions. And Dr. Moench, writing in the *Journal of the American Medical Association* (March 17, 1934) says: ". . . . I have shown definitely that the vaginal activity is not an important factor but that the body temperature alone, other factors remaining the same, will kill all sperms [father-cells] in twenty-four hours or so. The limit is certainly not more than from thirty-six to forty-eight hours."

It is therefore concluded that the father-cells have a limited life-span. The limit is placed at forty-eight hours.

We now have three scientific facts: 1. That the egg is expelled from 12 to 16 days prior to menstruation; 2. That the ovum (egg) cannot be fertilized after it is 24 to 48 hours old; 3. That the father-cell (spermatozoön) loses its power of fecundation within forty-eight hours.

Considering these three facts we may say that, in the case of a healthy woman with a regular menstrual cycle, or with an irregular menstrual cycle within certain known limits, the time when she can conceive and the time when she cannot conceive, between menstruations, are determined. For pregnancy does not occur at random—at any time, depending on a whim of fate. Nature is organized and orderly; she does not work haphazardly. Astronomers can predict to a second when a comet will appear or an eclipse will begin. Chemists know what happens when two chemicals are fused under certain known conditions. We all know from observing the movements of the sun, the earth, the moon and the stars that Nature operates in orderly cycles. These examples can be repeated at great length. And pregnancy, too, is due to cycles of Nature and is not accomplished in a hit-or-miss manner, as man has thought for ages. To quote Miller: "Pregnancy is not a hit-and-miss affair, but is regulated by the meeting of the egg and sperm cell before one or the other has withered and died." We know that there is a definite time in a woman's cycle of menstruation when the egg is present for only a few hours, and that at this time, *and this time only,* it is possible for a father-cell, which has a life of usefulness for forty-eight hours or less, to accomplish its destiny—namely, fertilizing the egg, or creating the state of pregnancy. At all other times the woman is sterile, and during these times she may indulge in the act of physical union without being apprehensive of ensuing pregnancy.

Therefore, by abstaining from cohabitation during the period of ovulation, husband and wife can exercise their marital rights, confident that a pregnancy will not occur. The opposite, also, is true. If the time of ovulation is the time when pregnancy occurs, then those wishing children will find it the most favorable time to cohabit in order to start pregnancy. Based on these known and proved scientific facts the arrival of children can be spaced, and parents can have or not have children as their health, economic status, and parent hunger dictate.

CHAPTER III

WHY MENSTRUATION?

Menstruation (the catamenia, monthly sickness, etc.) is a discharge of blood and mucus from the generative tract of the human female, and occurs periodically from puberty until the "change of life." Each menstrual flow is the culmination of a rhythmic or cyclic process in which the lining of the womb is prepared for the imbedding and attachment of a fertilized ovum. During the menstrual life of a woman she is capable of becoming pregnant. It has been said that menstruation is evidence of a disappointed womb, or is ". . . . merely a violent demolition of the premenstrual uterine edifice some days after the tenant [the fertilized egg] fails to appear."

Probably no other natural function of the body occupies the mind of a married woman so much as the anticipated arrival or cessation of this discharge. Throughout the ages it has been the basis of tribal laws and superstitions. Until a century ago there were many who believed that the moon exercised a control over its periodicity. Dr. Mead, an English physician famous in the eighteenth century, wrote on the effects of the moon on menstruation. Even today many laymen harbor fantastic ideas concerning this natural phenomenon in the mature female. How often do we hear that the cessation of the menses will lead to physical decline, tuberculosis, heart trouble and insanity? The intelligent know that organic diseases and pelvic disorders sometimes affect and increase or stop the monthly flow, but that the cessation of the flow does not cause these physical ills. Likewise there are today women who erroneously imagine that if their ovaries or womb were removed and menstruation ended, the blood that the body wants to throw off every so often would go to the brain and lead to mental derangement.

Menstruation is a natural function. It is an intimate part of the intricate process of ovulation, the formation of the corpus luteum, and the fertilization of the egg or (alternatively) the failure to become pregnant.

In the United States and Canada the age of the beginning of menstruation has been placed at fourteen years. Engleman arrived at this conclusion from the data of 20,000 cases. This writer found very little variation in the onset of menstruation in women living between Hudson Bay and the Gulf of Mexico. We once thought that climate played a big part in the time at which maturity begins, but this belief has now given way to the thought that race plays a more important role. Thus, we learn that the negresses of Somaliland begin to menstruate at sixteen, though one would imagine that the age would be much earlier. On the other hand, the Indians of the Arctic regions mature at twelve and a half; if climate exercised any influence, maturity in these girls would be past the age of fifteen years. In India menstruation begins in the fairly young, the first pregnancy often occurring at the early age of twelve years. In addition, many other factors exert an influence. Nutrition, surroundings, economic agencies, heredity, etc., retard or hasten the process. The girl who lives a life of ease, surrounded by every comfort and luxury, is likely to mature earlier than her poorer sister who is forced to work long hours in unhygienic surroundings and to eat foods of low caloric value.

It takes about a year for menstruation to become established. After a girl matures the first menstruations are irregular and the duration varies. Once her type becomes established she usually menstruates regularly, according to a fixed schedule. The great majority of healthy women flow regularly, they will tell you they "come on the dot"—the cycle becomes fixed. Whether or not a woman flows every twenty-one, twenty-eight, thirty or thirty-five days is not important. It is the periodicity of the flow that concerns the physician. When a woman has menstruated for years according to a fixed, regular rhythm, should she suddenly change her type something unusual has happened to her. Nature does not suddenly change established processes without a very good reason. Some women are irregular from the date of establishment. Therefore, every woman is peculiar unto herself as regards her periods. The time interval between the periods, if regular, has little bearing on this subject of biologic contraception, but whether or not the flow is regular in rhythmic cycles is important.

The duration of the flow varies in different women. The cycle established, a woman can usually time the duration of her flow. One woman in health may flow but two days while another woman may flow seven days. The periods, as a rule, last for four or five days. Roughly, any woman who menstruates for less than two days or more than seven may be considered abnormal. The amount of the flow varies in different individuals. For practical purposes a sudden increase or decrease in amount from what has been the customary habit is of more importance than the actual amount of blood lost. The flow usually is scanty at first and reaches its acme on about the second day. It is not unusual for menstruation to become suspended for twenty-four hours or more, after which it will return and continue its normal course.

Bleeding from the womb is not the only symptom of menstruation. In most women, for several days prior to the expected flow, certain premonitory symptoms are often present, such as pelvic pain or discomfort, backache, pains in the thighs, headaches, gastric upsets, more or less general malaise, excitability of temper, mental depression, and irritability, while in some certain skin eruptions appear. The woman learns to recognize these symptoms and evaluate them. These symptoms may continue during the first one or two days of the flow. In addition, she may experience irritability of the bladder and possibly burning urination. Just prior to menstruation the pulse-rate, the temperature, and the blood-pressure are slightly elevated. During the period these fall below normal, but once menstruation is over with they quickly return to the normal level. The severity of the symptoms of the menses varies and is experienced even by healthy women. Only a small percentage of women pass through this period without some discomfort or suffering; some of them become semi-invalids while menstruating.

Menstruation may be influenced to some extent by psychic excitement; this is especially true of fright and anxiety. Sudden news of a shocking nature may delay the flow. To quote Graves: "In women who menstruate normally the flow after having started may be suppressed by a sudden nervous shock, or such a shock may bring on the menses out of the regular time. It is a common experience in a gynecologic clinic that women whose periods are usually regular menstruate out of time under the mental excitement of waiting for operation. Menstruation is often delayed for several days or even a week in women who are laboring under fear of impregnation, and also in women who, being extremely anxious to become pregnant, have their minds tensely concentrated on the function." Many physicians have noted that an unusual mental upset causes a woman to miss her menstruation, and it may not appear again until her next regular date.

Menstrual blood usually does not clot, a peculiar phenomenon that is thought to be due to the presence of a ferment in the glands of the lining of the womb. However this has not been settled. The clotting of menstrual blood is evidence that an abnormal condition is present.

We speak of the menstrual cycle. This is because in health the average woman menstruates on certain fixed dates. This cycle has been divided into various phases. If we are to understand the subject of this book, we should learn something about these phases.

The phases of the menstrual cycle are determined by the changes in the mucous membrane lining the cavity of the womb. These phases are: 1. Menstruation; 2. State of regeneration; 3. The interval or resting stage; 4. Premenstrual stage or stage of congestion.

During the menstrual phase, the destructive changes in the glands of the lining of the womb and its blood-vessels cause a shedding of the entire spongy and compact portions of the mucosa. The flow contains red and white blood corpuscles, degenerated surface cells, vaginal and womb secretions, and many microörganisms, some of them disease-bearing. Menstruation may be said to be an exfoliation of the lining of the womb. The amount of the discharge varies. Hippocrates put the amount lost at 20 ounces, von Haller at 6 to 12 ounces, Smellis at 4 ounces, and Baudelocque at 3 or 4 ounces. As a matter of fact, it is difficult to estimate this accurately.

Just after menstruation the lining of the womb is

quite thin. The newly generated cells are very low but get higher as time goes on. The glands become straight or slit-like. This stage following menstruation, the post-menstrual phase or stage of repair, occupies about four or five days. By a gradual transition it passes into the next phase—the stage of quiescence, or interval stage.

The interval stage lasts about ten days to two weeks. Gradually, as this stage continues, congestion begins. The glands change to a slightly tortuous form and become wider. Later on these changes increase: the glands become wider and more tortuous, but there is no evidence of secretion.

Gradually the pregravid, premenstrual or secretory phase begins. This is the stage of preparation. The lining of the womb begins to be prepared to play host to an anticipated fertilized ovum. The lining of the womb becomes thick and velvety. There is an increase in the tissues and of the blood-supply. The activity of the glands of the womb increases. The womb may be likened to a bird building a nest: it is preparing a place for the fertilized ovum. When the egg begins its journey word is sent to the womb to make a room ready for the egg, should the egg become fertilized on the way. If it is fertilized, word is sent by the corpus luteum and a real bed (decidua) is prepared. Menstruation normally ceases during the pregnant state. If, however, the egg does not meet with a spermatozoön and become fertilized, word to this effect is sent to the uterus, and it proceeds to throw off the bed it has been preparing. This is menstruation. And so, month after month, this process continues: menstruation, repair, a resting stage, ovulation, the preparing of a bed for the fertilized ovum (which if it is not fertilized causes the bed to be cast out)—and the whole affair started over again. A rhythmic, regular process and each part of the cycle can be more or less accurately timed, though there are no clear lines of demarcation between the different phases.

Thus, we have a general idea of what Nature provides that man may continue the species.

The menstrual function continues for about thirty-five years. It is the reproductive period of a woman's life. Just as menstruation begins in the young girl so it ends in the woman, usually while she is in the late forties. When a woman stops menstruating she is at the climacterium or "change of life." Webster, many years ago, was responsible for the statement, "in temperate countries the menopause takes place in about 50 per cent of women between forty-five and fifty; in 25 per cent, between forty and forty-five; in 12½ per cent, between thirty-five and forty; and in 12½ per cent, between fifty and fifty-five." These figures are for the normal woman.

Today many authorities say 85 per cent reach the menopause in the late forties.

The change of life is apt to appear late if the age of puberty was early. Childbearing is said to have an influence on the time of the menopause. Bearing children tends to make the change come later. A woman's social status probably has little bearing on the matter, although it is claimed that the hard-working classes change earlier than those who have lived lives of leisure. Obesity and the cessation of menstruation were once thought to be related as cause and effect, but today we know that the obesity that appears at the time of menopause and the cessation of menstruation are both due to some condition of the ductless glands.

Some of the laity have an idea that the change of life is a perilous and critical time in a woman's life; a time potent with danger. In the average healthy woman it causes about as much upset as does the occurrence of puberty in the young girl. A woman is no more likely to become insane at this time than at any other time of her life. Many believe that abnormal bleeding (hemorrhage) at this time is a good thing, since it prevents the blood from going to the head. This is a serious misconception. Excessive and prolonged bleeding at the menopause may be a dangerous symptom, calling for medical advice.

The cessation of menstruation is but one of the symptoms of the change of life. To the woman, however, it is the symptom of chief importance. Some women dread the time when they will "change," while others welcome it, feeling that after the menopause they will have their "best days."

Some women cease menstruating abruptly for all time, but as a rule it is a gradual process. The woman suddenly skips one, two or three periods; then, menstruation appears again. As time passes the interval between the periods lengthens. The duration of the flow becomes shorter. Finally a permanent cessation of menstruation ensues, and we say the woman has "gone through the change of life."

A prominent symptom, often sufficiently annoying as to make life nearly unbearable, is "hot flushes." This is a vasomotor disturbance and usually involves the head, neck and upper part of the chest. In some women the hot flushes are mild and infrequent. In others they may be frequent—as many as fifteen or twenty-five a day—and often continue during the night. The patient's head and neck, and possibly her upper chest, become bright red and hot, and the woman feels suffocated. A flush is usually of short duration. It may be followed by a profuse sweat. When a flush is present the woman hungers for cool air, and often, even during the coldest days of winter, she will throw open a window and stand near it, while experiencing this annoying symptom. Often the flushes are frequent at night, thereby disturbing the woman's sleep, and making her weary, nervous and irritable.

The "flashes of heat," like the "hot flushes," are difficult of explanation. They usually occur as hot tingling waves, which may affect the whole body. They come quickly but go just as quickly. Often the woman sweats independently of the hot flushes or the flashes of heat.

At the menopause, women usually have a moderate rise in blood pressure. Also, at this time, dizziness is quite common. Some women have attacks of fainting. Headaches may be persistent and make the woman's life miserable. These are usually vertical, situated at the back of the head. Palpitation of the heart is not uncommon, as are attacks of a "fast, racing heart," probably caused by the associated effect of the menopause upon the thyroid.

The sensation of itching may be persistent and very troublesome at this time. At times, this itching may cover the entire body, while at other times it may be confined to the genitalia.

At the beginning of puberty the girl is irritable and her nervous system is unstable. The same is true of the end of full development. The woman is easily upset, irritable, and may be given to periods of depression.

Gastro-intestinal disturbances occur at this time. But the menopause does not occasion gall-bladder disease, gall-stone formation, stomach ulcers or tumorous growths. In both sexes this age is the time when these ills are most likely to occur.

During the change of life various forms of skin eruptions are common. Hives may be of frequent occurrence and persistent. The same is true of acne.

The permanent cessation of the menstrual function has no effect upon the *libido sexualis,* or sexual desire

It is not diminished—in fact, it may be markedly increased.

Currier offered some good common-sense advice when he wrote, "All that tends to develop and strengthen the physical part of woman—to render her insensitive to the ordinary ills of life, to make her forgetful of self—is favorable to a normal menopause."

The period of fecundity over, the ovaries become markedly diminished in size, and they take on a "peach-stone" appearance. Active follicles are no longer seen, or the corpus luteum, because ovulation has ceased and forever. The womb shrinks to one-half or one-third its normal size.

Some women have odd conceptions concerning the possibility of pregnancy at this time of life. They speak of "change of life babies," or will tell you that it is impossible to become pregnant about the time of the menopause, or that it is then that a woman is most likely to become impregnated. Many women, who have for years practised caution (whatever this means) or some form of birth-control, at this period cease such precautions, thinking themselves safe, and become pregnant. Once the menopause has been completed, pregnancy is impossible, but as long as ovulation continues just that long is pregnancy possible. A woman can become pregnant during the menopause, though the chances are against this happening.

The duration of the menopause varies. Some women go through quickly, in less than a year's time. Others suffer symptoms for three to five years. Schroeder, after a study of the problem, put the normal time at 1.11 years. However, many American workers think this too short and say that a year and a half to two years is nearer the truth.

We have written this chapter not because it has a close bearing on the safe and unsafe periods in a woman's menstrual cycle, but because so many women have no conception of what menstruation is all about. We feel that the reader, now that she has some knowledge of puberty, ovulation and menstruation, will be better equipped to grasp thoroughly the principle of the sterile and the fertile periods, and thus to learn how to defer or space pregnancy.

CHAPTER IV

MOTHERHOOD

MATRIMONY is an institution intended for the conservation of the race. Biologically speaking, the cardinal goal of a married woman is to become a mother. When man was a nomad and the tribe a law unto itself, the number of children and the rapidity of successive births gave neither parent much thought or concern. In fact, for a long period in the history of primitive man, the reason for a woman's becoming pregnant was unknown. It was thought that when the gods looked with favor on a woman they evidenced their beneficent will by getting her with child. It was not dreamed that intercourse between the sexes was responsible for this condition. Male and female cohabited and never realized that it served to do more than satisfy a hunger. But if a woman pleased the "spirits" then it was thought she was rewarded by becoming a mother: and it was not noted that a virgin never had offspring. It was supposed that she had neglected to live up to the very letter of some superstitious custom, and so had displeased the spirits, who accordingly frowned on her and kept her sterile.

But the time came when man emerged out of the darkness and gradually learned the truth. The face of the world, also, changed. Villages, towns, and cities arose on the plains and in the hills. The mode of barter became intricate. A thing called money began to be used. Families no longer followed the sun and grass so that their cattle might graze, or engaged in the hunt so that they themselves might have food. The word "economic" took on a practical meaning. In some instances large families became a burden. The science of medicine went through a long and slow evolution. For hundreds of years it was in the doldrums, until not so many centuries ago it became a science as well as an art. Physicians learned that pregnancy was not always a normal, physiological thing. Often it jeopardized the health, perhaps even the life, of the woman. Science looked for a way to stop or defer pregnancy. But to do either was against certain religious laws. The orthodox or devout would not break these ecclesiastical laws and therefore had children, often in rapid succession, and whenever the mother paid the price for her family by becoming an invalid or dying, people could only murmur that "it was God's will." After all, there may be some truth in this explanation. But there has never been a law of God or man that people have not tried to evade or break. Thus hundreds of years ago, man attempted to prevent conception.

There is no need to dwell on the methods advocated. None were perfect. Millions walk this earth who are in a sense the result of an artificial contraceptive that failed in its purpose. As stated, reliable statistics prove that modern birth-control methods are slightly over 93 per cent effective. The methods advocated by proponents of artificial birth-control have been and are condemned by the Catholic Church and other Christian bodies. In no circumstances may their followers use any artificial method to prevent conception and there are other religious bodies that hold similar views. Nor has medicine formally approved these methods. In many localities it has been unlawful to give contraceptive information or to sell contraceptives. Yet millions of women and men have secretly resorted to these methods, that they might regulate the births of their children, though anyone who has done this knows that, apart from all religious scruples, they are unnatural and messy, and offend the sense of the esthetic. Moreover, certain mechanical devices have caused pelvic infection, invalidism, even death.

As an easy way out the majority of physicians, when urged by their patients, will consent to impart birth-control knowledge, but these same physicians know how often such methods fail, usually in the case of women who really have a valid reason for wishing to defer pregnancy for a time. Until Ogino and Knaus offered a natural method of biologic contraception man had to resort to these artificial means.

But the vast majority of married women hunger for children. Many normal, healthy women dream of marriage, and of the children they will bring into the world. For this reason we shall consider in this chapter the subject of sterility, pregnancy, and the most opportune time for pregnancy to occur.

To many, pregnancy seems a miracle, and it truly is. Nothing is more fascinating than to consider the intricate processes of Nature in transforming a cell of microscopic diameter into a pink, crying, healthy baby.

At best, we can here discuss only the high-lights, since the average layman would soon be lost in a maze of scientific explanations should we attempt the average text-book descriptions.

Let us begin with the sterile ovum just entering the Fallopian tube. This egg has but a short time to be discovered by a mate and fertilized. As we know, the life of an ovum is short, not much longer than a day; this has superseded the older view, now definitely disproved, which held that the life-span of the ovum is about two weeks.

Just as the ovum is entering the tube as a result of the marriage-union, some two hundred million father-cells are deposited on and about the neck of the womb. Many millions of these father-cells are killed or die in the genital tract. A great many wriggle their way through the opening into the womb and hurry on to the tubes, each one hunting for the ovum. Maybe theirs is the instinct of self-preservation. For the spermatozoön that fertilizes the ovum becomes a part of the ovum which, in turn, becomes the baby. The other millions of father-cells, failing in their quest, perish.

Once it was thought that in man, as in some of the lower animals, spermatozoa may retain their potency for many days. The evidence now seems quite certain that they lose their capacity to fertilize the egg in about one or two days, though their motility (their power to move) may continue longer.

The ovum lives about a day unless fertilized. The father-cells have a life-span of three days, at the longest. We continue to repeat these facts, for a reason.

The ovum is in one of the Fallopian tubes. Spermatozoa also are in that tube, and soon the ovum is surrounded by them. One father-cell gets to the ovum ahead of the others. The head of the father-cell immediately begins to enter the ovum. After the head has entered the egg, the tail rapidly disappears, and in a short time nothing is left of the original father-cell. The ovum is now fertilized; the woman is now pregnant; a new human being is in the making, and the sex of the child and all of its future physical and racial characteristics are determined. All this usually happens somewhere in the third of the tube farthest from the womb.

After the head of the father-cell is in the egg it swells up and becomes a typical nucleus. It then approaches and fuses with the nucleus of the ovum. The resulting cell begins to grow and to divide. In the nuclei that fuse are little flecks of viscid protoplasm. These flecks are so small as to be hardly discernible with a high-powered microscope. They are called chromosomes.

They are the bearers of hereditary destiny. Each human is what he is because of the particular outfit of chromosomes with which he is equipped. The only connection between one generation and the next is found in the germ cells, and whatever is inherited is carried in these cells.

The cells divide by a process called cell-division or segmentation. By this process of cell-division growth occurs.

The fertilized egg proceeds on its journey to the womb, propelled by the action of the cilia (hair-like filaments) of the tube, and aided by the peristalsis (worm-like movements) of the tubal muscles.

Meanwhile, word has been sent to the womb to make ready for an important guest. The increase in the structures that takes place in the premenstrual or congestive stage of the menstrual cycle goes on, and a bed or decidua is formed. At this time the womb lining is thicker, velvety, soft, spongy and rich in blood-vessels.

It takes about seven or eight days for the fertilized egg to reach the cavity of the womb. Once there, the egg selects or happens to reach a favorable spot and becomes embedded. Usually it sinks into this bed lining the womb. After it becomes embedded many curious and wonderful things happen. Cells that have an arrosive action eat into the muscular lining of the womb, and in these places the beginning of a placenta or afterbirth is formed and takes root.

Meanwhile the cell-division continues, the primary layers are formed, and from these layers the various structures of the foetal body are built. From a cell the mass becomes an embryo and so grows into a foetus, to be expelled, at the end of pregnancy, a fully formed baby.

The foetus lies inside a balloon-like structure filled with fluid. This bag is composed of membranes in close apposition to the lining cavity of the womb. The foetus floats in this fluid chamber.

The placenta or afterbirth is a vascular organ resembling a flat cake. The umbilical cord leading to the child (connected at its navel) is attached to the placenta. The mother's blood flows in and around the placenta and through the cord to the child. In this way the child is nourished. The child's blood flows back through the cord to the placenta, carrying off waste-products.

When fertilized, the ovum is but a microscopic cell. A little later it can just be seen. In two weeks it has increased to the size of a small bean, and in four weeks it is as large as a walnut. At eight weeks it may be said to be as large as a lemon, and at sixteen weeks it is the size of a baseball. At nine months, or "term," the womb is about the size and shape of a watermelon. The child, floating in the liquid in the sac, moves and changes its position. After the mother "feels life"— about halfway through her pregnancy—the child makes rhythmic, jerky movements. These often become very active and may be so active as to disturb the mother's rest.

At the end of ten lunar months (or about nine calendar months) the child is at "full term" or "ripe," and ready to be born.

Out of a clear sky, the mother notices that she urinates more frequently, has a vaginal discharge and begins to experience slight, intermittent cramp-like pains, due to the contractions of the womb. She may note a slight vaginal bleeding. She is now in labor and about to give birth. The intervals between the pains get shorter; the duration and intensity of the pains longer and greater. The child is born. It takes a breath into its lungs. It cries. Another human being, the result of the meeting of an ovum and a father-cell, joins his fellows on this earth.

Many women marry and long for babies but do not become pregnant. When a woman has been married for two years, has not attempted to prevent conception by unnatural means, and has lived a normal married life, it may be assumed that she is sterile. This is a problem that engages the full time, attention, and skill of some physicians. Nothing brings a greater thrill to the woman, her husband, and the physician than for her to become pregnant, after a long period of sterility that has called for medical tests, treatments, and even, at times, surgical interference.

This is not the proper place to go into the finer points of this subject. We must assume, for our purposes, that the woman is normally built and therefore regularly ovulates healthy eggs; that the man is healthy and that his father-cells are alive and capable of impregnating or fertilizing the ovum. They have been married for some time and pregnancy has not occurred. In this discussion we are concerned only with the most favorable time for cohabitation so that pregnancy may ensue.

Later on we will learn how to apply the facts we have now at hand, and be able to figure the sterile and fertile periods in a given woman's menstrual cycle.

There are times when pregnancy will not occur as a result of physical union. Likewise, there are times most propitious for pregnancy to occur.

If the facts we have reviewed are founded on scientific truths and we can do no more than accept them, because they have been discovered and checked by men of integrity and sound scientific standing—then the principle of the fertile time is simple of interpretation. As has been said, this theory works like a two-edged sword. If we can determine a safe, sterile time when intercourse will not result in pregnancy, then we can determine also the time at which it *will* so result

CHAPTER V

HOW TO APPLY THE MODERN METHOD OF BIRTH CONTROL

IN ORDER to make this subject clearer a few common examples will be cited. But the reader who would follow this method can eliminate most of the mathematics *by turning to the diagrams* given further on in this book and fitted to *each particular case*.

Let us assume that you are a woman married for about a year. So far you have not become pregnant. You are in good health. There are no apparent reasons why pregnancy should not be possible. Your menstruation is of the 28-day type, and this has been your regular habit for several years; seldom has there been a variation of more than a day one way or the other. This is the way in which you will reckon the days on which you have the best chance of becoming pregnant.

We know, from Ogino's and Knaus' studies, that ovulation takes place from 12 to 16 days prior to the next expected menstruation. We know that the female cell or ovum lives a day or less. In your case, therefore, if intercourse has occurred on the last possible day of ovulation, unless impregnation has taken place at this time, then the ovum cannot be fertilized during this cycle. So the limit of your ovulation time *ends* with the 12th day prior to your next menstruation. (Note that you count backwards from the next, expected menstrual period.)

But ovulation may begin as early as 16 days before the expected menstruation. The father-cells may live as long as 3 days. The life span of the father-cell is usually two days, in exceptional cases three days; so, to be absolutely safe, we use the three-day period. Therefore, if you had intercourse 1, 2 or 3 days prior to the first possible day of ovulation it would be possible for you to become pregnant. Example: It is March first. On March 2nd intercourse occurs. On March 5th, the fertile period begins. Assume that the father-cells live their possible full 3-day life span. On the last day of their life-span ovulation takes place. Fertilization occurs and you become pregnant. We therefore add 3 days to the ovulation time for this possibility.

In the woman with a 28-day menstrual cycle, as has been said, the ovulation period is from 12 to 16 days *prior* to the next menstruation. Inasmuch as the father-cells may live 3 days we must add these days to the 16-day period, making it 19 days. This makes the period when pregnancy is possible from 12 to 19 days prior to the first day of the next expected period.

The above figuring always dates from the *first* day of the next expected period. The duration of the actual menstrual flow has nothing to do with determining the safe and unsafe periods.

On the next pages simple examples are given to show how to apply your calendar to the *Modern Method*.

FOR THE WOMAN WHOSE PERIODS ARE REGULAR

Place your calendar before you.

Determine the date on which your next menstrual period starts. Count *back* or subtract 19 days. (A) On that date your fertile or unsafe time will *start*. (B) Now, stop and count *forward* or add on 7 more days from this date and you come to the *end* of your fertile of unsafe time.

In the days between (A) and (B) *inclusive,* pregnancy is probable. At all other times during the monthly cycle it is improbable.

Example:

Assume that you expect to menstruate on October 29th. (A) Count back 19 days and you come to October 10th. That is when the fertile time begins. (B) Add on 7 more days and you arrive at the 17th. That is when the fertile or unsafe time ends. Pregnancy is probable from the 10th to the 17th *inclusive*. It is improbable on any other day in the monthly cycle.

OCTOBER

SUN.	MON.	TUE.	WED.	THU.	FRI.	SAT.
	1	2	3	4	5	6
7	8	9	~~10~~	~~11~~	~~12~~	~~13~~
~~14~~	~~15~~	~~16~~	~~17~~	18	19	20
21	22	23	24	25	26	27
28	29	30	31			

FOR THE WOMAN WHOSE PERIODS ARE
IRREGULAR

Place your calendar before you.

Determine the *first* possible date of the next menstrual period. Count *back* or subtract 19 days. (A) On that date your fertile or unsafe time will *start*. (B) Now, stop and count *forward* or add on 7 more days *plus* the number of days of possible lateness and you come to the *end* of your fertile or unsafe time.

In the days between (A) and (B) *inclusive,* pregnancy is probable. At all other times during the monthly cycle it is improbable.

Example:

For the woman whose monthly cycle varies from 26 to 30 days, we will assume that her last menstrual period started on October 3rd and her *earliest* expectant date to menstruate is October 29th. (A) Count back 19 days to October 10th. That is when the fertile time begins. (B) Add on 7 more days *plus* the 4 days of possible lateness and you arrive at the 21st. That is when the fertile time ends. Pregnancy is probable from the 10th to the 21st *inclusive*. It is improbable on any other day in the monthly cycle.

OCTOBER						
SUN.	MON.	TUE.	WED.	THU.	FRI.	SAT.
	1	2	3	4	5	6
7	8	9	10	11	12	13
14	15	16	17	18	19	20
21	22	23	24	25	26	27
28	29	30	31			

This method is the simplest way to figure the safe and unsafe periods unless you use the charts in the following pages. In the charts for irregular periods we count back from the *latest* probable starting date for the next period, instead of the earliest. This is done in order to show the longest possible cycle and does not change the result in any way.

A point that is sometimes confusing is that in the case of a woman with a short menstrual cycle—for example, the 21-day type—her fertile period starts on the 3rd day after the beginning of the menstruation. If this woman menstruates for three or four days how would she figure her safe time and her unsafe time? For the woman with a short (say 21-day) cycle we must assume that the fertile period begins on the 3rd day after menstruation starts. Unless she has stopped menstruating before that 3rd day, then—if she does not want to become pregnant —she will have to wait until the end of the fertile period before she can safely have intercourse. On the other hand, if she does want to become pregnant, the woman with a 21-day cycle ought to have intercourse on any of the days between the 3rd and 10th after the beginning of her menses.

For the woman who does not wish to figure this out for herself, we have arranged diagrams in Chapter VI covering all the most common types of menstrual cycles. The fertile period as marked on each woman's diagram is the time when she is most likely to conceive. Her sterile period is likewise shown.

We would not give the impression that, in a woman who has been unable to conceive, all she has to do is to make sure she cohabits during her period of fecundity and that within no time she will be rewarded by becoming pregnant. We repeat that, all the other factors (and there are many) being equal and normal, according to this theory the fertile period is the only period when pregnancy is possible. But unless she has been checked by a physician she cannot know whether all other factors *are* equal and normal. She may be a physically healthy woman and yet her womb may never have grown to its full size. If her womb is of this decidedly infantile type, it may be the factor rendering her sterile. This is but one of many abnormalities that may be responsible for her continued sterility.

This theory is diametrically opposed to the common theory. It has been a favorite conclusion of the laity (and of many physicians) that the "dangerous" time—the time when a woman must be careful if she does not want to conceive—was just after and just before the menstrual dates. "Then," the average woman has reasoned, "halfway between my periods I must be safe." We know however, that this is actually the fertile time—somewhere during the middle of the menstrual cycle; and the "safe" times are usually just after, and *always* just before, the menstrual period, because these are the times of natural sterility.

If, every time an ovum emerged from its ovary, it became fertilized, the woman would be in an almost continuous state of pregnancy. But since there usually is an interval of some days between acts of intercourse, one can readily understand how an ovum may be freed, get into a tube and perish. From this, a woman might reason that if she has intercourse every day during her fertile period, the ovum would be sure to become fertilized. But Nature has placed a check-rein on this, also. Frequent intercourse—in the case of the average man— causes the father-cells to lose their virility, and they are not so likely to impregnate an ovum. For this reason it is possible for the woman who wishes to become pregnant to cohabit during the fertile period for several months before she gets her wish.

The woman who is truly sterile had better place herself in the hands of a competent physician who is conversant with these problems, and be advised by him.

CHAPTER VI

CHARTS OF NORMAL REGULAR MENSTRUATION: AND IRREGU-
LAR CYCLES VARYING BETWEEN ONE AND FOUR DAYS

SINCE THIS method of computing a woman's period
of fertility and sterility was discovered, thousands of
women have relied on it as a means of spacing the arrival
of their babies, or have followed it, for one reason or
another, in order to prevent conception. The method
has a wide vogue in Europe, where it has been applied
for several years. It is beginning to become known in
this country. It has been predicted that within a short
time it will be the method of choice among the majority
here.

Many people do not have mathematical minds, and
it is common knowledge that many women cannot
"figure." At best, reading a description of the various
methods by which the fertile and sterile days may be
computed will perhaps leave some confused. Others
may continue to make some common error in their
figuring, which may lead to disappointment or tragedy.

Although we have attempted in simple language to
explain the basis for this theory leading to the final
conclusions, and have tried to explain several ways to
figure each particular case, we realize that, after all, each
woman is interested only in her particular problem,

Above all else, she wants to know accurately the exact time of her sterile and fertile period in her particular menstrual cycle.

Errors in determining the fertile and the sterile periods in a menstrual cycle are serious errors. With this in mind, in an effort to help the reader to reckon accurately, we have offered the following charts. They represent every regular menstrual cycle from, 21 to 35 days; also irregularities of the cycle up to four days. From these charts, at a glance, the fertile and sterile periods may be seen.

To select her particular chart, a woman must know her type of menstruation, so as to identify the chart that covers her case. For example, she menstruates irregularly from 28 to 31 days, and she therefore turns to the chart for this cycle.

If a woman has been menstruating regularly and then begins to vary, even though only one day, she should consult the chart showing that variation or irregularity period. Inasmuch as many may vary in their menstrual cycles it is important to keep a written record of menstrual dates. Calendars are supplied (Chap. VIII) for this purpose.

In this chapter we do not repeat the method of computing the sterile and fertile times. We have *printed in red* the *fertile days,* or the days when pregnancy is possible. *The days printed in green are sterile days,* or days when marital union will not cause pregnancy.

These are *menstrual charts, not* calendars. The day

at the beginning of the circle marked in black is always the first day of menstruation.

Therefore, should a woman wish to know the time most propitious for her to become pregnant, her particular chart will show, at a glance, her days of fertility, during which the marital act is most likely to result in the ovum's becoming impregnated.

On the other hand, should she wish not to become pregnant, she will abstain during the time of fertility. She will have marital relations only on the days of sterility. These are the "safe" days.

For the timid, or those who wish to take every extra precaution, it is suggested that another day be added at the beginning and the end of the period of fertility. *This is not necessary, however.* Above everything else follow the laws laid down. Otherwise, failure may ensue. If failure results because of carelessness, or "taking a chance," or lack of coöperation between husband and wife, it is not the fault of the method, but is the fault of the individual.

The following charts are of normal, regular menstrual cycles. The first chart is of the 35-day cycle. A day is taken off on each succeeding chart of the menstrual cycle until the 21-day cycle has been reached.

The days in red are days of fertility. At this time pregnancy is possible.

The days in green are days of sterility. At this time pregnancy is not possible.

35 DAY CYCLE

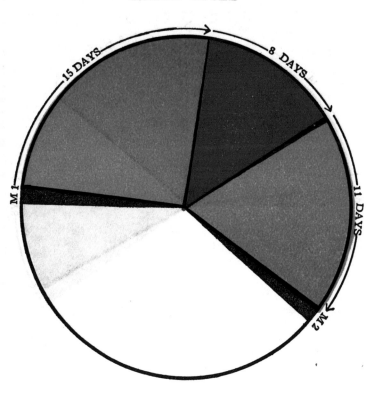

● Fertile or Unsafe Days.
● Sterile or Safe Days.
M 1—Day when *last* menstrual period *started.*
M 2—Day for *next* menstrual period to *start.*

34 DAY CYCLE

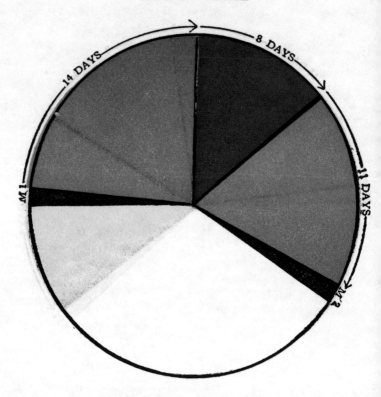

●   Fertile or Unsafe Days.
●   Sterile or Safe Days.

M 1—Day when *last* menstrual period *started*.

M 2—Day for *next* menstrual period to *start*.

33 DAY CYCLE

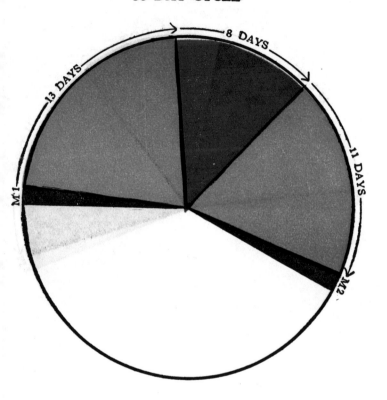

● Fertile or Unsafe Days.
● Sterile or Safe Days.
M 1—Day when *last* menstrual period *started*.
M 2—Day for *next* menstrual period to *start*.

32 DAY CYCLE

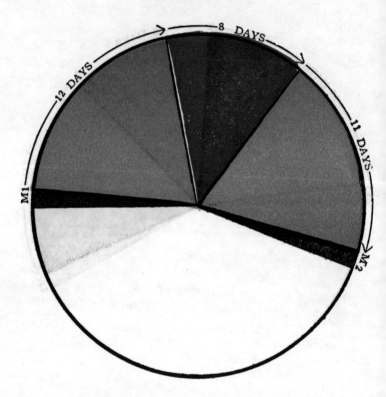

● Fertile or Unsafe Days.
● Sterile or Safe Days.
M 1—Day when *last* menstrual period *started*.
M 2—Day for *next* menstrual period to *start*.

31 DAY CYCLE

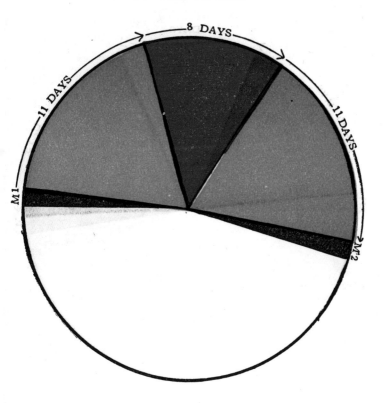

- 🔴 Fertile or Unsafe Days.
- 🔵 Sterile or Safe Days.

M 1—Day when *last* menstrual period *started*.

M 2—Day for *next* menstrual period to *start*.

30 DAY CYCLE

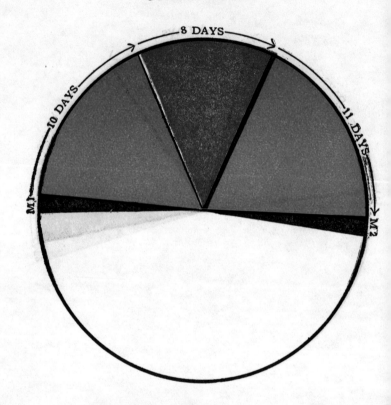

Fertile or Unsafe Days.
Sterile or Safe Days.
M 1—Day when *last* menstrual period *started*.
M 2—Day for *next* menstrual period to *start*.

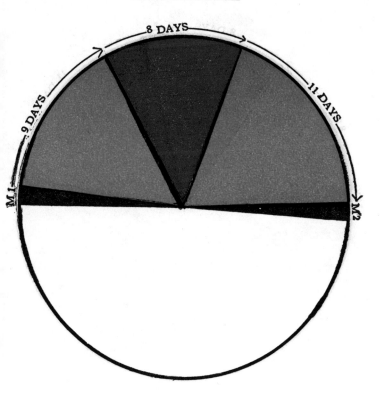

29 DAY CYCLE

8 DAYS

9 DAYS

11 DAYS

M 1

M 2

● Fertile or Unsafe Days.
● Sterile or Safe Days.

M 1—Day when *last* menstrual period *started.*
M 2—Day for *next* menstrual period to *start.*

28 DAY CYCLE

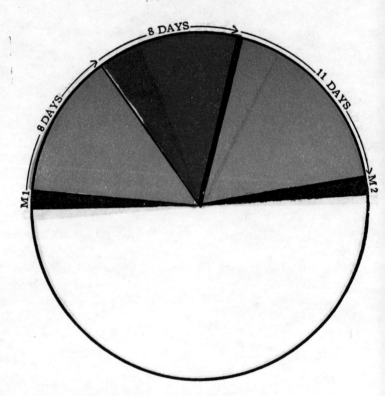

● Fertile or Unsafe Days.
● Sterile or Safe Days.
M 1—Day when *last* menstrual period *started*.
M 2—Day for *next* menstrual period to *start*.

27 DAY CYCLE

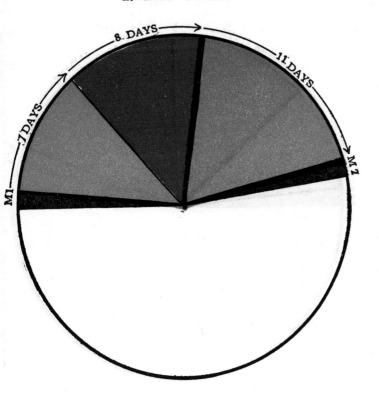

● Fertile or Unsafe Days.
● Sterile or Safe Days.
M 1—Day when *last* menstrual period *started.*
M 2—Day for *next* menstrual period to *start.*

26 DAY CYCLE

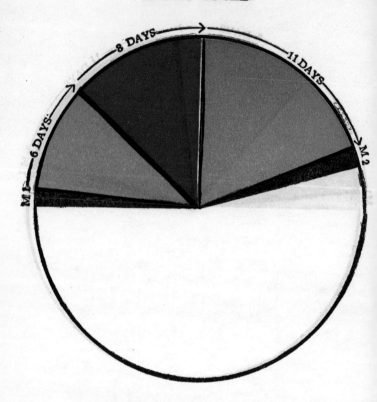

● Fertile or Unsafe Days.
● Sterile or Safe Days.
M 1—Day when *last* menstrual period *started*.
M 2—Day for *next* menstrual period to *start*.

25 DAY CYCLE

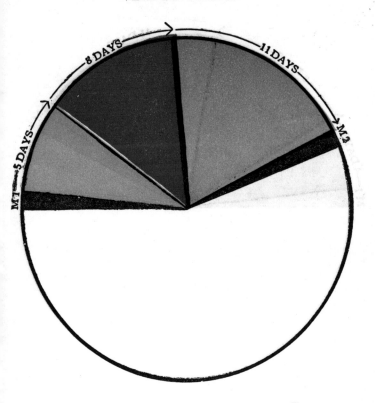

8 DAYS

11 DAYS

M 1 — 5 DAYS

M 2

● Fertile or Unsafe Days.
● Sterile or Safe Days.
M 1—Day when *last* menstrual period *started.*
M 2—Day for *next* menstrual period to *start.*

24 DAY CYCLE

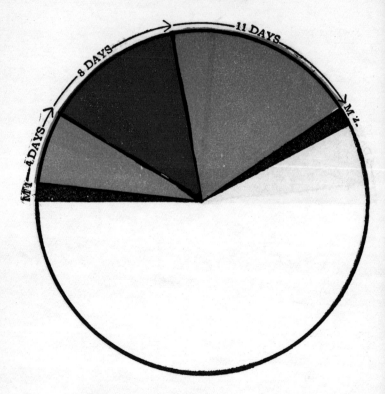

● Fertile or Unsafe Days.
● Sterile or Safe Days.
M 1—Day when *last* menstrual period *started*.
M 2—Day for *next* menstrual period to *start*.

23 DAY CYCLE

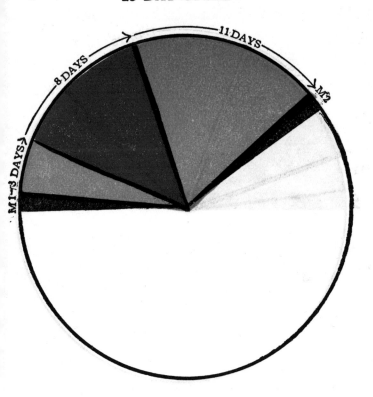

11 DAYS

8 DAYS

M 1—3 DAYS

M 2

● Fertile or Unsafe Days.
● Sterile or Safe Days.
M 1—Day when *last* menstrual period *started.*
M 2—Day for *next* menstrual period to *start.*

22 DAY CYCLE

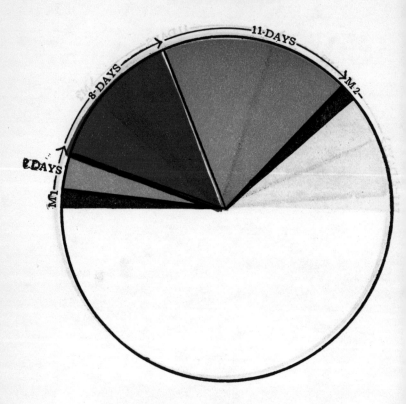

Fertile or Unsafe Days.
Sterile or Safe Days.
M 1—Day when *last* menstrual period *started*.
M 2—Day for *next* menstrual period to *start*.

21 DAY CYCLE

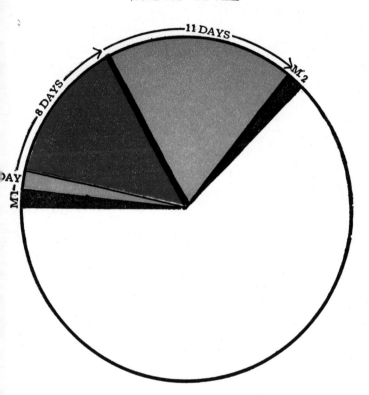

Fertile or Unsafe Days.
Sterile or Safe Days.
M 1—Day when *last* menstrual period *started*.
M 2—Day for *next* menstrual period to *start*.

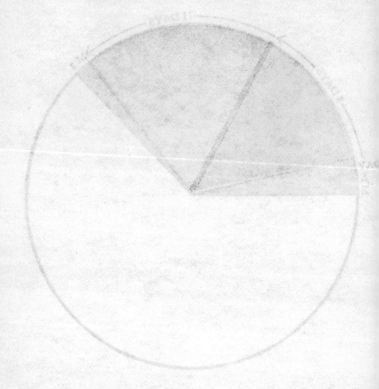

Fertile or Unsafe Days
Sterile or Safe Days
M 1—Day when the menstrual period started.
M 2—Day for a new menstrual period to start.

The following charts are of menstrual cycles of a 1-day irregularity.

The days in red are days of fertility. At this time pregnancy is possible.

The days in green are days of sterility. At this time pregnancy is not possible.

34–35 DAY CYCLE

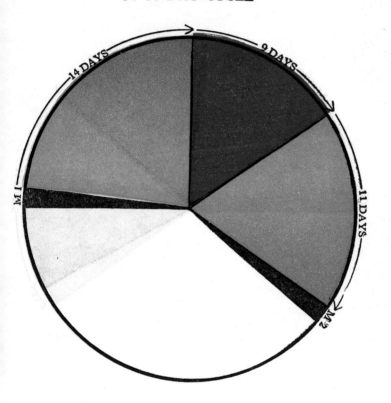

● Fertile or Unsafe Days.

● Sterile or Safe Days.

M 1—Day when *last* menstrual period *started.*

M 2—Latest day for *next* period to *start.*

33–34 DAY CYCLE

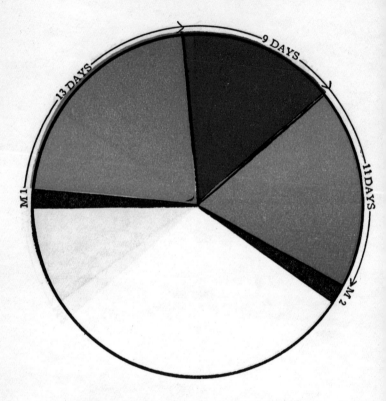

- Fertile or Unsafe Days.
- Sterile or Safe Days.

M 1—Day when *last* menstrual period *started.*

M 2—Latest day for *next* period to *start.*

32–33 DAY CYCLE

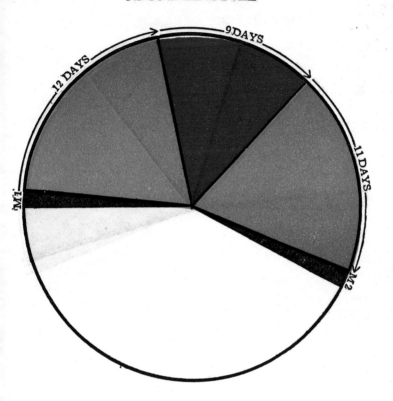

Fertile or Unsafe Days.
Sterile or Safe Days.

M 1—Day when *last* menstrual period **started**.
M 2—Latest day for *next* period to *start*.

31–32 DAY CYCLE

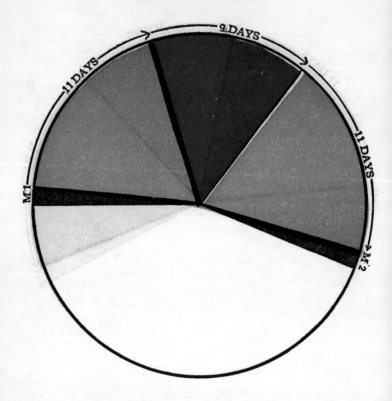

● Fertile or Unsafe Days.
● Sterile or Safe Days.
M 1—Day when *last* menstrual period *started.*
M 2—Latest day for *next* period to *start.*

30–31 DAY CYCLE

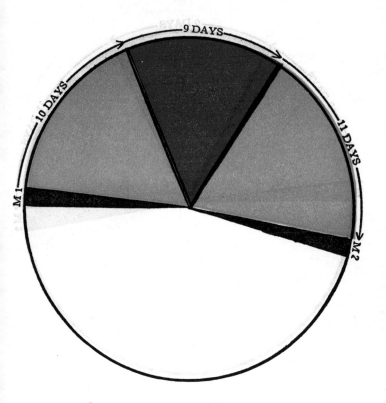

● Fertile or Unsafe Days.
● Sterile or Safe Days.
M 1—Day when *last* menstrual period *started.*
M 2—Latest day for *next* period to *start.*

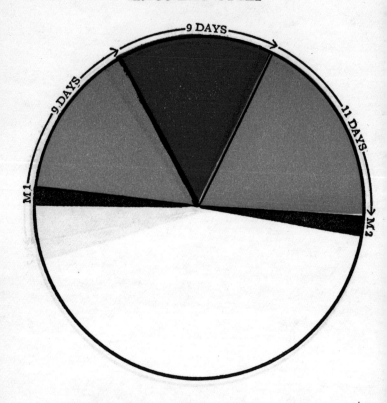

· 29–30 DAY CYCLE ·

9 DAYS

9 DAYS

11 DAYS

M 1

M 2

● Fertile or Unsafe Days.
● Sterile or Safe Days.
M 1—Day when *last* menstrual period *started*.
M 2—Latest day for *next* period to *start*.

28–29 DAY CYCLE

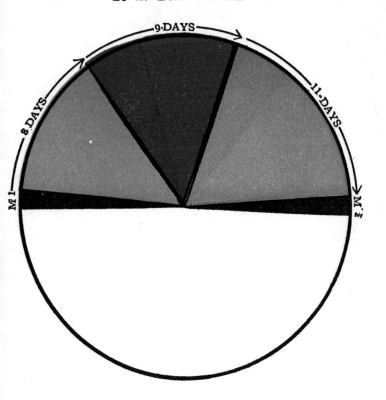

● Fertile or Unsafe Days.
● Sterile or Safe Days.
M 1—Day when *last* menstrual period *started*.
M 2—Latest day for *next* period to *start*.

27–28 DAY CYCLE

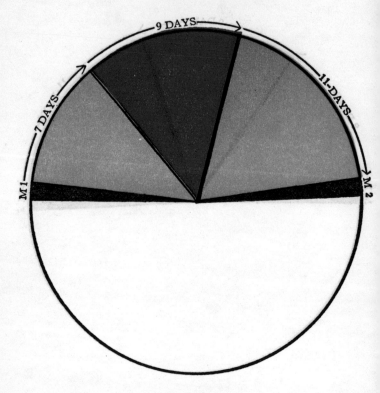

● Fertile or Unsafe Days.
● Sterile or Safe Days.
M 1—Day when *last* menstrual period *started*.
M 2—Latest day for *next* period to *start*.

26–27 DAY CYCLE

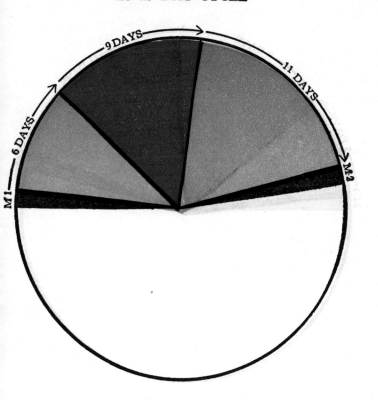

● Fertile or Unsafe Days.
● Sterile or Safe Days.
M 1—Day when *last* menstrual period *started.*
M 2—Latest day for *next* period to *start.*

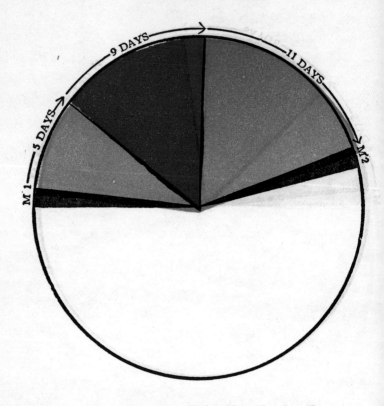

'25–26 DAY CYCLE

9 DAYS

11 DAYS

5 DAYS

M 1

M 2

● Fertile or Unsafe Days.
● Sterile or Safe Days.
M 1—Day when *last* menstrual period *started*.
M 2—Latest day for *next* period to *start*.

24–25 DAY CYCLE

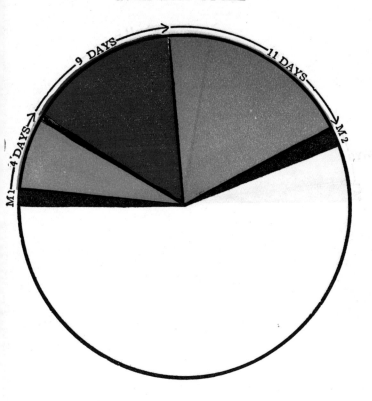

● Fertile or Unsafe Days.
● Sterile or Safe Days.
M 1—Day when *last* menstrual period *started.*
M 2—Latest day for *next* period to *start.*

23–24 DAY CYCLE

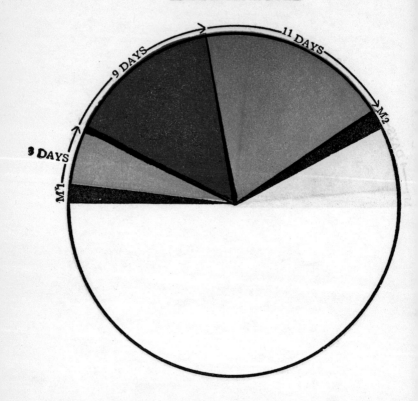

11 DAYS

9 DAYS

3 DAYS

M 1

M 2

● Fertile or Unsafe Days.
● Sterile or Safe Days.
M 1—Day when *last* menstrual period *started.*
M 2—Latest day for *next* period to *start.*

22–23 DAY CYCLE

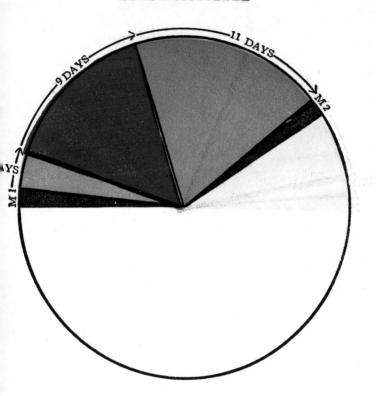

● Fertile or Unsafe Days.
● Sterile or Safe Days.
M 1—Day when *last* menstrual period *started*.
M 2—Latest day for *next* period to *start*.

21–22 DAY CYCLE

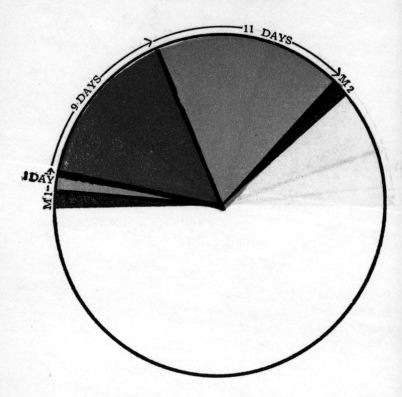

Fertile or Unsafe Days.
Sterile or Safe Days.
M 1—Day when *last* menstrual period *started.*
M 2—Latest day for *next* period to *start.*

The following charts are of menstrual cycles of a 2-day irregularity.

The days in red are days of fertility. At this time pregnancy is possible.

The days in green are days of sterility. At this time pregnancy is not possible.

33 TO 35 DAY CYCLE

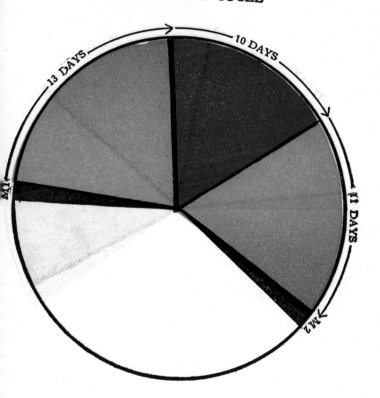

● Fertile or Unsafe Days.
● Sterile or Safe Days.
M 1—Day when *last* menstrual period *started.*
M 2—Latest day for *next* period to *start.*

32 TO 34 DAY CYCLE

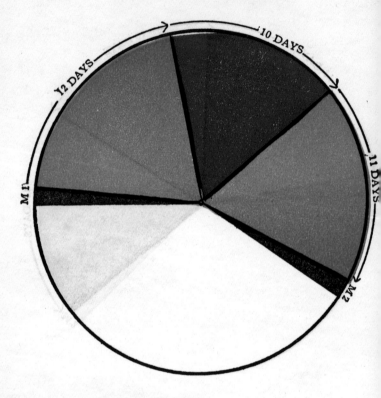

● Fertile or Unsafe Days.
● Sterile or Safe Days.
M 1—Day when *last* menstrual period *started*.
M 2—Latest day for *next* period to *start*.

31 TO 33 DAY CYCLE

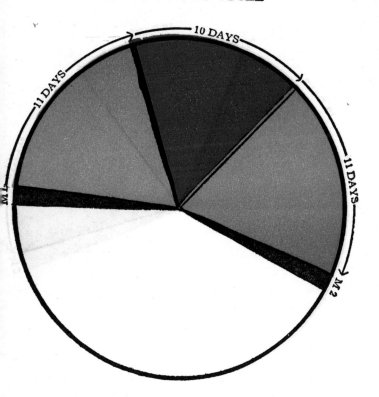

● Fertile or Unsafe Days.
● Sterile or Safe Days.
M 1—Day when *last* menstrual period *started*.
M 2—Latest day for *next* period to *start*.

30 TO 32 DAY CYCLE

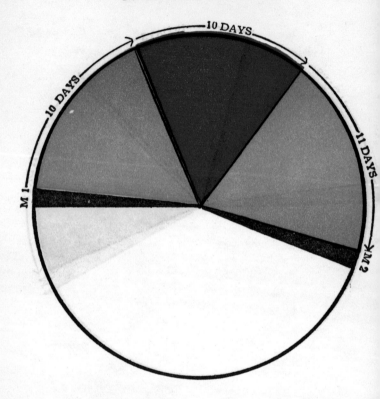

● Fertile or Unsafe Days.
● Sterile or Safe Days.
M 1—Day when *last* menstrual period *started*.
M 2—Latest day for *next* period to *start*.

29 TO 31 DAY CYCLE

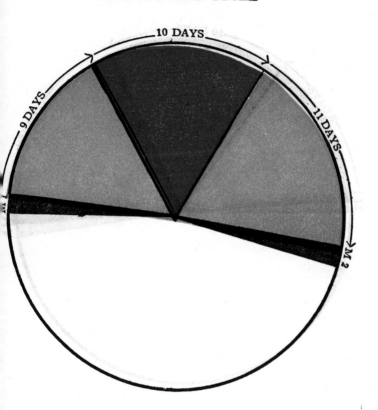

● Fertile or Unsafe Days.
● Sterile or Safe Days.
M 1—Day when *last* menstrual period **started.**
M 2—Latest day for *next* period to *start*.

28 TO 30 DAY CYCLE

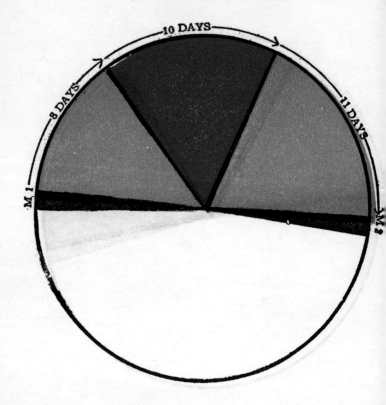

● Fertile or Unsafe Days.
● Sterile or Safe Days.
M 1—Day when *last* menstrual period *started*.
M 2—Latest day for *next* period to *start*.

27 TO 29 DAY CYCLE

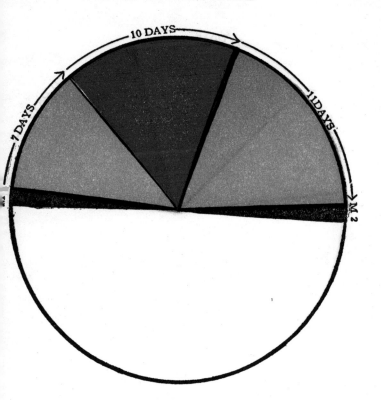

- **Fertile or Unsafe Days.**
- **Sterile or Safe Days.**

M 1—Day when *last* menstrual period *started*.
M 2—Latest day for *next* period to *start*.

26 TO 28 DAY CYCLE

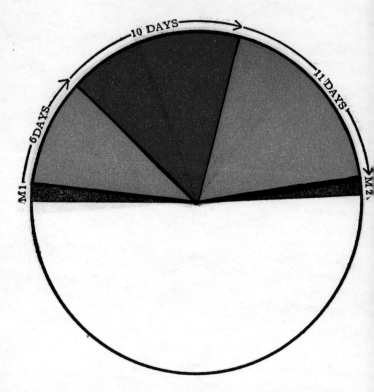

Fertile or Unsafe Days.
Sterile or Safe Days.
M 1—Day when *last* menstrual period *started.*
M 2—Latest day for *next* period to *start.*

25 TO 27 DAY CYCLE

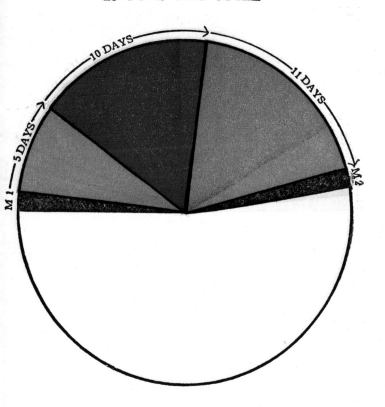

● Fertile or Unsafe Days.
● Sterile or Safe Days.
M 1—Day when *last* menstrual period *started*.
M 2—Latest day for *next* period to *start*.

24 TO 26 DAY CYCLE

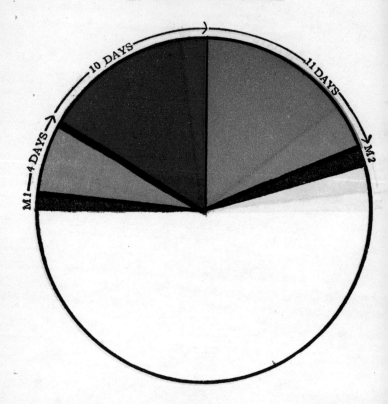

● Fertile or Unsafe Days.
● Sterile or Safe Days.
M 1—Day when *last* menstrual period *started*.
M 2—Latest day for *next* period to *start*.

23 TO 25 DAY CYCLE

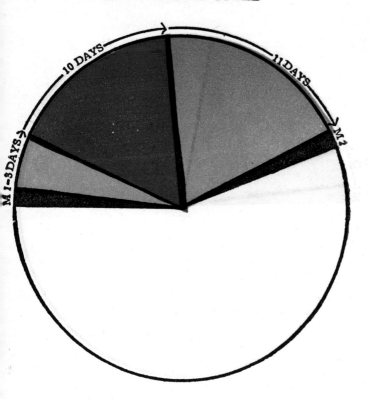

● Fertile or Unsafe Days.
● Sterile or Safe Days.
M 1—Day when *last* menstrual period *started*.
M 2—Latest day for *next* period to *start*.

22 TO 24 DAY CYCLE

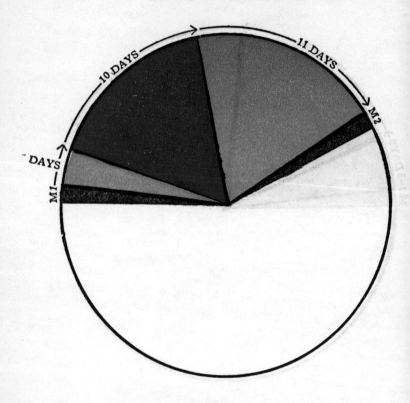

● Fertile or Unsafe Days.
● Sterile or Safe Days.
M 1—Day when *last* menstrual period *started.*
M 2—Latest day for *next* period to *start.*

21 TO 23 DAY CYCLE

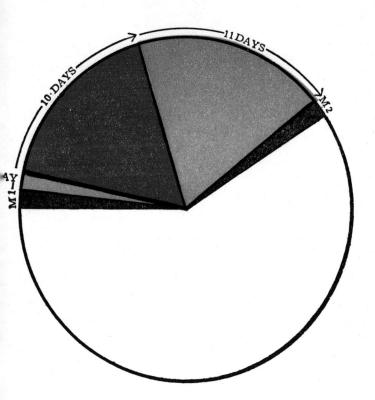

● Fertile or Unsafe Days.
● Sterile or Safe Days.
M 1—Day when *last* menstrual period *started*.
M 2—Latest day for *next* period to *start*.

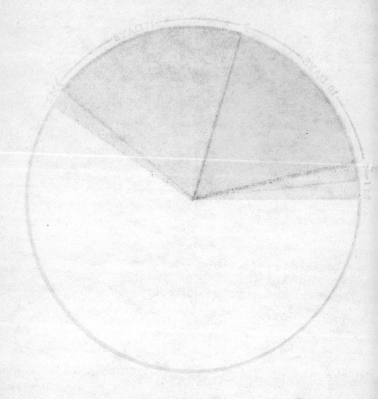

Fertile or Unsafe Days

Sterile or Safe Days.

M 1—Day when last menstrual period began.

M 2—Latest day for next period to start.

The following charts are of menstrual cycles of a 3-day irregularity.

The days in red are days of fertility. At this time pregnancy is possible.

The days in green are days of sterility. At this time pregnancy is not possible.

32 TO 35 DAY CYCLE

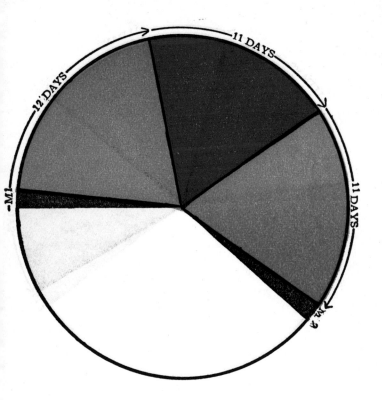

● Fertile or Unsafe Days.
● Sterile or Safe Days.
M 1—Day when *last* menstrual period *started*.
M 2—Latest day for *next* period to *start*.

31 TO 34 DAY CYCLE

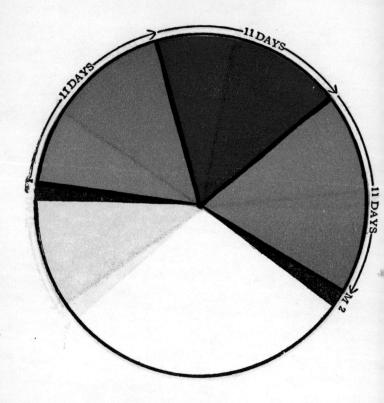

● Fertile or Unsafe Days.
● Sterile or Safe Days.
M 1—Day when *last* menstrual period *started*.
M 2—Latest day for *next* period to *start*.

30 TO 33 DAY CYCLE

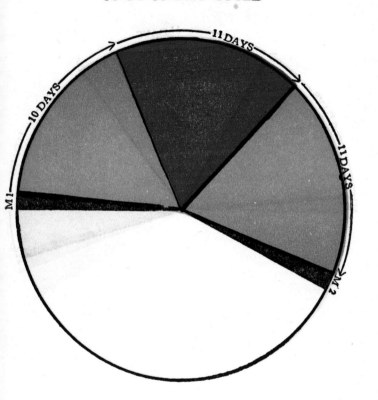

- ● Fertile or Unsafe Days.
- ● Sterile or Safe Days.

M 1—Day when *last* menstrual period *started*.
M 2—Latest day for *next* period to *start*.

29 TO 32 DAY CYCLE

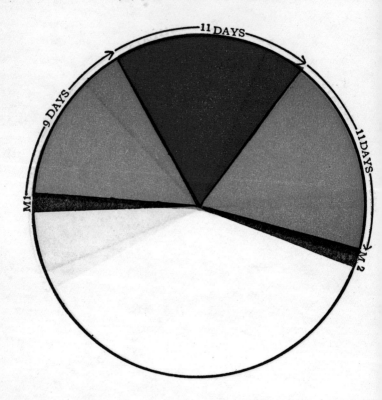

● Fertile or Unsafe Days.

● Sterile or Safe Days.

M 1—Day when *last* menstrual period *started*.

M 2—Latest day for *next* period to *start*.

28 TO 31 DAY CYCLE

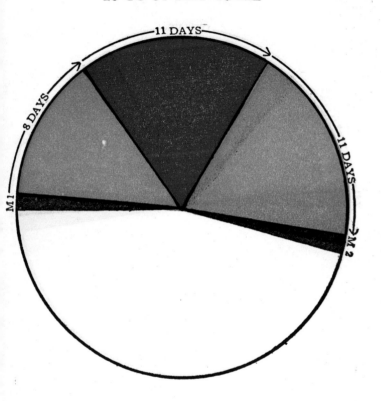

● Fertile or Unsafe Days.
● Sterile or Safe Days.
M 1—Day when *last* menstrual period *started.*
M 2—Latest day for *next* period to *start.*

27 TO 30 DAY CYCLE

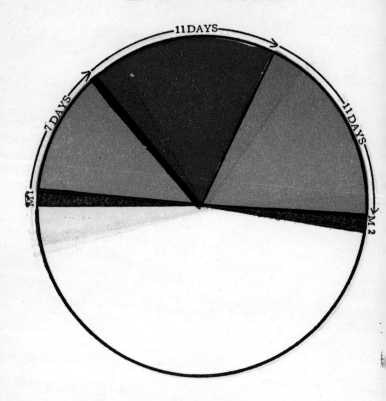

● Fertile or Unsafe Days.
● Sterile or Safe Days.
M 1—Day when *last* menstrual period *started*.
M 2—Latest day for *next* period to *start*.

26 TO 29 DAY CYCLE

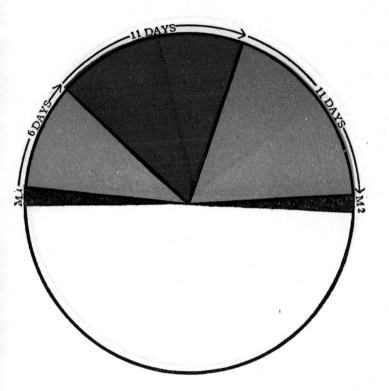

Fertile or Unsafe Days.
Sterile or Safe Days.
M 1—Day when *last* menstrual period *started*.
M 2—Latest day for *next* period to *start*.

25 TO 28 DAY CYCLE

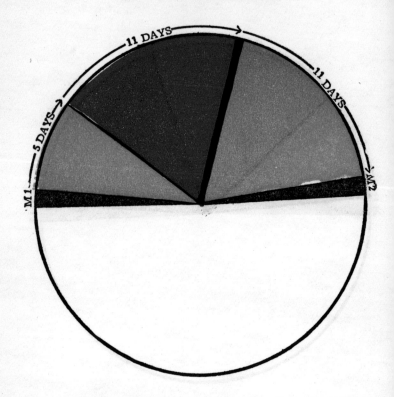

● Fertile or Unsafe Days.
● Sterile or Safe Days.
M 1—Day when *last* menstrual period *started*.
M 2—Latest day for *next* period to *start*.

24 TO 27 DAY CYCLE

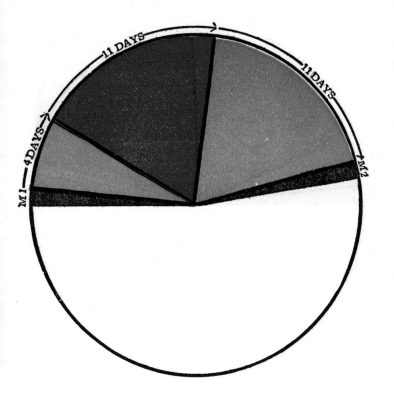

● Fertile or Unsafe Days.
● Sterile or Safe Days.
M 1—Day when *last* menstrual period *started*.
M 2—Latest day for *next* period to *start*.

23 TO 26 DAY CYCLE

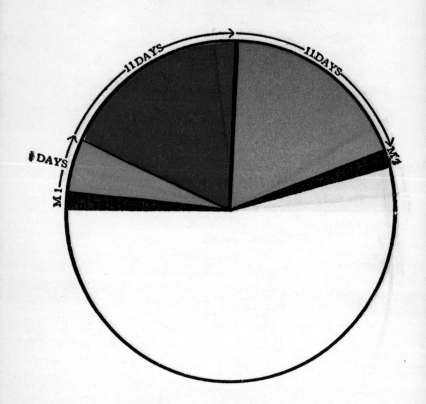

● Fertile or Unsafe Days.

● Sterile or Safe Days.

M 1—Day when *last* menstrual period *started*.

M 2—Latest day for *next* period to *start*.

22 TO 25 DAY CYCLE

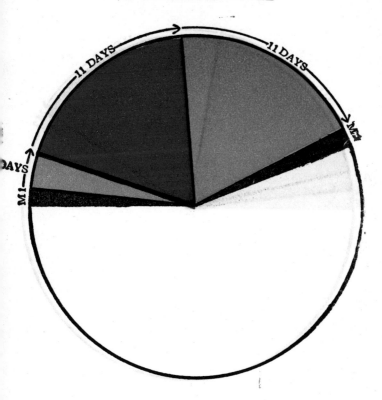

11 DAYS   11 DAYS

DAYS

M 1   M 2

- Fertile or Unsafe Days.
- Sterile or Safe Days.

M 1—Day when *last* menstrual period *started*.

M 2—Latest day for *next* period to *start*.

21 TO 24 DAY CYCLE

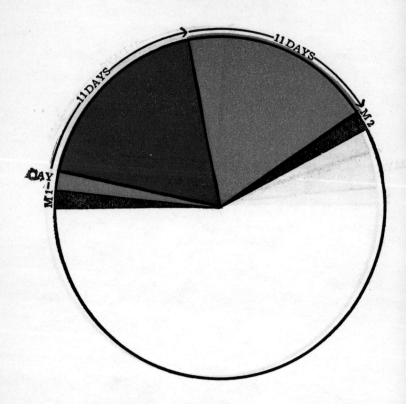

● Fertile or Unsafe Days.
● Sterile or Safe Days.
M 1—Day when *last* menstrual period *started*.
M 2—Latest day for *next* period to *start*.

CHARTS OF FOUR-DAY IRREGULAR CYCLES

The following charts are of menstrual cycles of a 4-day irregularity.

The days in red are days of fertility. At this time pregnancy is possible.

The days in green are days of sterility. At this time pregnancy is not possible.

31 TO 35 DAY CYCLE

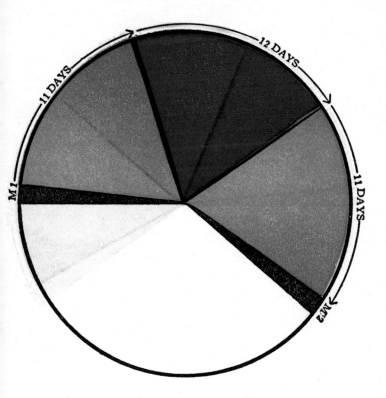

⬤ Fertile or Unsafe Days.
⬤ Sterile or Safe Days.
M 1—Day when *last* menstrual period *started*.
M 2—Latest day for *next* period to *start*.

30 TO 34 DAY CYCLE

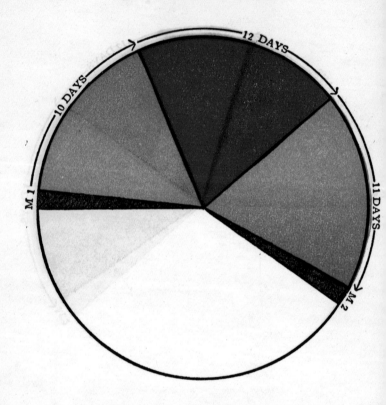

● Fertile or Unsafe Days.
● Sterile or Safe Days.
M 1—Day when *last* menstrual period *started*.
M 2—Latest day for *next* period to *start*.

29 TO 33 DAY CYCLE

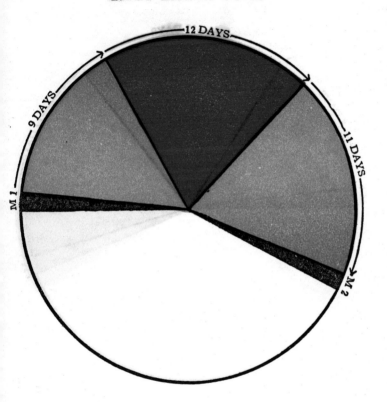

● Fertile or Unsafe Days.
● Sterile or Safe Days.
M 1—Day when *last* menstrual period *started*.
M 2—Latest day for *next* period to *start*.

28 TO 32 DAY CYCLE

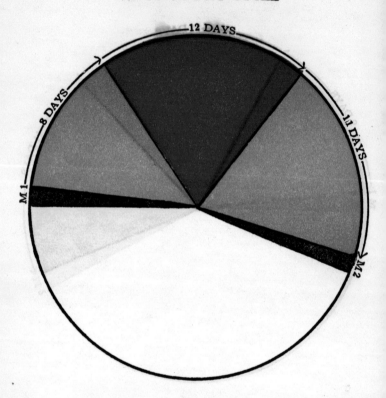

● Fertile or Unsafe Days.
● Sterile or Safe Days.
M 1—Day when *last* menstrual period *started*.
M 2—Latest day for *next* period to *start*.

27 TO 31 DAY CYCLE

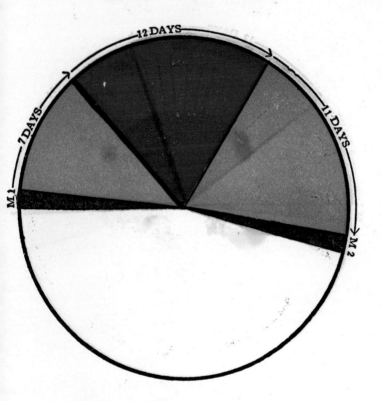

● Fertile or Unsafe Days.
● Sterile or Safe Days.
M 1—Day when *last* menstrual period *started.*
M 2—Latest day for *next* period to *start.*

26 TO 30 DAY CYCLE

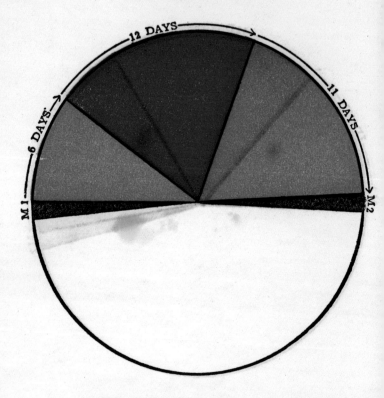

● Fertile or Unsafe Days.
● Sterile or Safe Days.
M 1—Day when *last* menstrual period *started*.
M 2—Latest day for *next* period to *start*.

25 TO 29 DAY CYCLE

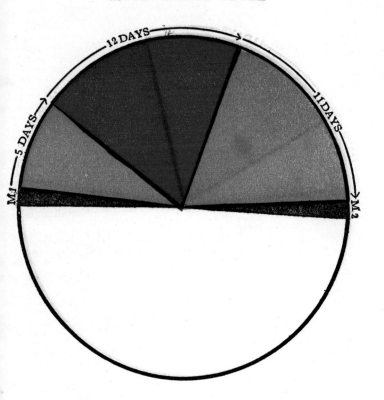

- **Fertile or Unsafe Days.**
- Sterile or Safe Days.

M 1—Day when *last* menstrual period *started*.

M 2—Latest day for *next* period to *start*.

24 TO 28 DAY CYCLE

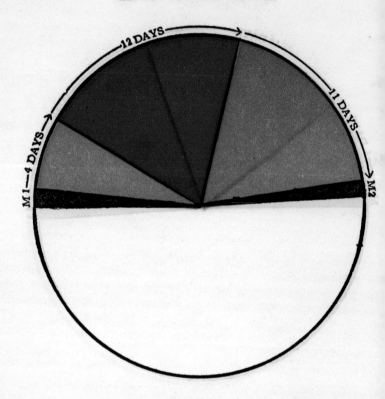

● Fertile or Unsafe Days.
● Sterile or Safe Days.
M 1—Day when *last* menstrual period *started*.
M 2—Latest day for *next* period to *start*.

23 TO 27 DAY CYCLE

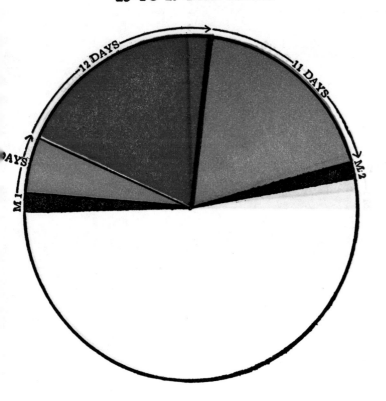

●   Fertile or Unsafe Days.
●   Sterile or Safe Days.
M 1—Day when *last* menstrual period *started.*
M 2—Latest day for *next* period to *start.*

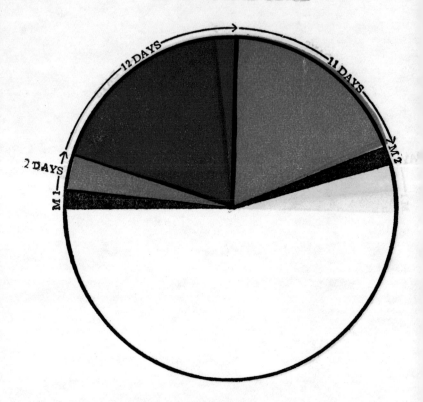

22 TO 26 DAY CYCLE

Fertile or Unsafe Days.
Sterile or Safe Days.
M 1—Day when *last* menstrual period *started.*
M 2—Latest day for *next* period to *start.*

21 TO 25 DAY CYCLE

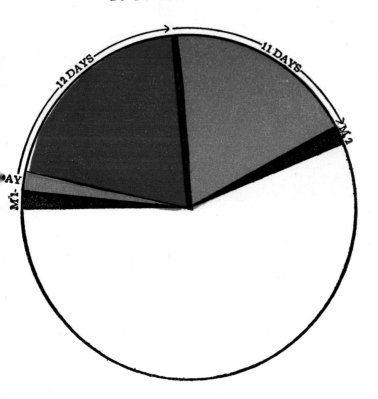

● Fertile or Unsafe Days.
● Sterile or Safe Days.
M 1—Day when *last* menstrual period *started*.
M 2—Latest day for *next* period to *start*.

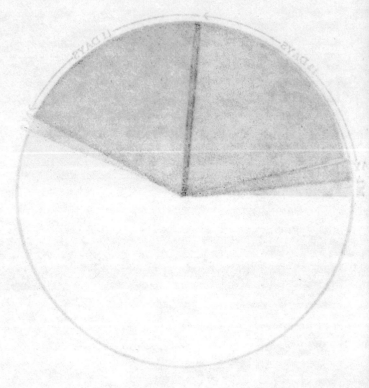

21 TO 25 DAY CYCLE

Fertile or Unsafe Days.

Sterile or Safe Days.

M 1—Day when last menstrual period started.

M 2—Latest day for next period to start.

SUMMARY

Eᴛʜᴇʀ ᴛʜᴇʀᴇ is a definite period of fertility fixed in the menstrual cycle of the average, healthy woman, and it is during this period of ovulation that pregnancy is possible, or the entire scientific structure upon which this theory is based is false, and the method is unreliable and worthless.

The foundations upon which this natural method of birth regulation are based are: 1. That the ovary expels an egg some time between 12 and 16 days before an expected menstruation. 2. That the egg has a short life-span, probably not more than 1 day. 3. That the father-cells may live 1, 2 or, possibly, 3 days.

Much work has been done in this country and abroad by eminent scientists in support of the above enumerated facts. The general conclusion is that the maximum time of fertility in the human female is on the day of ovulation.

Dr. Ogino, who, with Dr. Knaus, has been given the credit for bringing this method to the attention of the medical profession, kept detailed records of hundreds of women who had sexual relations only during the periods of sterility, and *not in one instance did pregnancy occur*. Other scientists have arrived at the same conclusions.

A sense of confidence in this method is created by the experiments conducted by Doctors A. D. Miller, C. H. Schulz, and D. W. Anderson, and reported in an article which appeared in the June, 1933, issue of *Surgery, Gynecology and Obstetrics* (the official organ of the American College of Surgeons). These physicians called for volunteers in order to prove or disprove the soundness of this new theory of pregnancy-control. Ninety-seven couples responded to the invitation. Examinations of all were made to detect any condition which might affect potency. All but five per cent of the volunteers were parents. Eight nationalities were represented. The women of the group gave histories of having twelve different types of menstrual cycles. Eighty-seven couples had normal marital relations 725 times during the prescribed *sterile* periods only, and *in each case not one pregnancy resulted*. Ten couples had sexual union during the prescribed period of *fertility,* and *in each case pregnancy resulted*. The writers' conclusions were:

"The sperm and egg cells detached from their respective breeding places have a very limited time to live. For the egg cell it is not longer than 1 day. For the sperm cell it is 2 to 3 days. Every normal regularly menstruating woman has a definite ovulation period. Every normal regularly menstruating woman has a definite period of physiological sterility and a definite period of fertility in each cycle. Cohabitation must be properly timed with ovulation if pregnancy is to result. Pregnancy may be brought about or avoided at will by the observation of these two periods of time."

Dr. J. M. Culligan, in an address before the Minnesota State Medical Association at Rochester (May 22, 1933) is reported to have said: "There is a definite time relation between ovulation and menstruation. The ovum is capable of fertilization only for a few hours. Spermatozoa remain fecund not longer than three days. There is, therefore, a fertile and a sterile period in women's menstrual cycle."

To a question directed to the editor of the *American Journal of Medicine* (July 22, 1933), the reply was: "The motility of sperms does not mean that such sperms have fertilizing properties. . . . Students are agreed that in the human species sperms are dead after twenty-four hours. . . . The unfertilized ovum is short-lived, according to the best evidence."

We read that a group of moralists, desiring to secure an impartial report of the value of Dr. Ogino's work, invited the eminent Dr. Raoul E. de Gouchteneere, of the Lambert Gynecological Institute, Brussels, to investigate, appraise and advise them concerning this new theory of the avoidance of conception. Dr. de Gauchteneere concurred in Dr. Ogino's findings, and in his report wrote: "We may thus conclude that the fertile period in each menstrual cycle does not exceed eight days . . . The numerous cases of practical application observed by Ogino, Knaus, Smulders, Georg and others have amply confirmed the correctness of these views. If medical opinion in general has been slow to accept them, the explanation is that it is difficult to abandon a theory which one has been accustomed to accept as definitive."

That sage and scholar, James J. Walsh, M.D., Ph.D., wrote: "Nature apparently intended that this law should be discovered in the course of time, when population was increasing rapidly, and then furnished the perfectly natural method by which would be brought about such limitation of birth as would keep the world from being overcrowded."

The old conception of the "unsafe time" was just before and after the menstrual periods. Today this conception must go into the mental wastepaper basket. Now, we know the times of fertility and sterility as worked out by scientists in many countries of the world.

If these premises are wrong, then scientists will have to discard most of their present-day teaching regarding ovulation, the action of the corpus luteum and menstruation.

There is little doubt that during the next few years an animated and acrimonious controversy will be waged concerning the pros and cons of this method. There will be some who refuse to accept the new teaching, no matter what proofs are offered in support of it. Certain commercial interests will feel a loss in revenue from the sale of contraceptives. Physicians who now earn large incomes by advising women how to prevent conception, and then by selling them a contraption with detailed instructions as to its use, will not welcome a method that calls for nothing but natural sex-relations, the only

stipulation being that if the couple do not desire conception to occur they *must abstain from sexual union*
during the period of fertility during each menstrual
cycle.

Contrary to the general impression, many physicians
have little or no faith in the value of any artificial
methods of contraception to date. Physicians have de-
livered full-term women of healthy babies that were
supposed to have been prevented by unnatural methods
or by the employment of all kinds of chemical substances or mechanical gadgets.

Of course nothing is perfect. And the freak case will
always turn up when least expected. We read of the
woman who has become pregnant without ever having
menstruated, or of the woman who had both ovaries
and tubes removed and later on gave birth to twins;
medical literature abounds in the unusual. But for all
sane purposes we must accept the ninety-nine per cent
as against the rare one per cent. Worth-while medical
discoveries are applied to the large majority of common,
usual cases.

Reports of reliable men in this field of work indicate
that the various artificial birth-control methods fail in
from seven to ten per cent of all cases, whereas, from
reports available of the efficacy of Nature's modern
method of control, we learn that failures have been
reported in only about three per cent. In all fairness,
allowing for exaggeration on the part of all the interested parties, let us suppose that all methods are equal

in value. To date the proponents of the Ogino-Knaus method claim far superior results; but let us suppose that one method is no better than the other. On this assumption who, in the name of common sense, would invest in a chemical paste, a powder or a liquid, or a mechanical contrivance, or resort to unnatural relations, when by following Nature's way of avoiding conception all that is required is natural physical union at certain times in each menstrual cycle? The answer is obvious.

We know of a woman who said she knew all about the new method but would not follow it because "using a contraceptive gives one a sense of security while this new method seems too simple to be true." This woman is twenty-seven years old and has had six children and two miscarriages. One of the hardest things to do is to change established habits.

When these facts permeate the minds of the women of this country, a subject which has caused controversy among physicians, churchmen, and laity will be closed. Either this method will be the method of all normal, refined women, or it will fall because of the number of its failures. There can be no middle ground. It is, or it is not, a reliable, sure method. Among those in foreign countries and in this country who have conducted clinical tests in large numbers of people, the evidence to date is overwhelmingly in its favor.

Many mechanical devices or abnormal practises detract from propriety in the marriage union and tend to cheapen or lower the act.

Gynecologists, almost as a unit, have condemned the practice of inserting certain mechanical devices into the neck of the womb. These devices so employed have caused pelvic infection, peritonitis, and even death. Moreover, chemicals employed in various forms in the generative tract have caused serious reactions. In many instances these have made the victims invalids, unable to fulfill their marital responsibilities, and there have been reported in medical literature cases of death following the use of such substances in this manner. We are told that fly-by-night concerns are selling the public certain contraceptives "of no more value than water."

The Catholic Church and many other Christian bodies have been unalterably opposed to artificial birth-control. In many localities it is considered a crime to impart birth-control knowledge or information to the healthy, or to sell artificial contraceptives. Organized medicine has never endorsed artificial birth-control. At present, there are committees of physicians who have undertaken a study of the various means of artificial birth-control with the object of reporting at a future date regarding what means are best and safest in their opinion. It has been realized that many artificial contraceptives have been advertised that in themselves are a menace to health.

Dr. H. Sutherland is responsible for this statement: "Contraception is unphysiological because, apart from preventing pregnancy, it inhibits far-reaching physiological process." And Dr. E. Heinrich says, "These measures [artificial contraceptives] are dangerous to health."

The patriarch of American gynecology is Dr. Howard A. Kelly of Baltimore. Long ago (October 16, 1915) in *Harper's Weekly,* writing of birth-control, he affirmed: "Practically, I find that people who come to me having used various mechanical devices for preventing conception have lost something in their married life which ought to have been more precious to them than life itself."

Dr. Frederick J. McCann, in his book *The Effect of Contraceptive Practices on the Female Sexual Organs,* wrote: "All methods of contraception are harmful to the female. They only differ in being more or less so. . . . When the female is deprived of the nutritional value of spermatic fluid by methods of contraception, both local and general changes are produced in her body." Finally, Dr. Edith Harper claims that "contraceptive methods are offensive to persons of refined dispositions."

Owing to the present-day vogue of making birth-control topics newspaper items, women may get the idea that all physicians believe in and endorse these artificial, unnatural methods. We have quoted from articles of several leaders in their field in order to dispel such an error. Of course, not all physicians agree with those who go to extremes and see nothing but great harm resulting from the use of all contraceptives; but the majority of physicians know that some methods are not entirely devoid of the possibility of being harmful, and that in many instances the user is doomed to disappointment in the end.

The *Modern Method,* intended for the *avoidance* of pregnancy, is not truly a method of *prevention.* *Nothing* is *used* or *done to prevent conception.* Sexual union is indulged in normally. The woman lives and practises a normal sex life. But, since she knows that certain days of her menstrual cycle are days of fertility, she abstains from sexual relations on any of those days if she wishes to avoid conception. Should she desire to become pregnant she has intercourse during her period of fertility, knowing that this is the time when pregnancy is possible. Thus she has children when she desires.

Dorothy Dunbar Bromley, in *Harper's Magazine,* October, 1934 (Birth Control and the Depression), quotes Dr. Eric M. Matsner, Medical Director of the American Birth Control League, who says, "The method [modern method] is doomed to failure when applied to the type of woman most frequently seen at contraceptive clinics, the type who cannot depend upon the coöperation of her husband." Both husband and wife must play the game together and fairly in order to attain the ends desired. Unless both parties coöperate failure will result. Again, the method will not be the cause of failure but the participating partners.

What is the attitude of the Roman Catholic Church regarding this natural method?

The Catholic Church always has been and is unalterably opposed to artificial birth-control. If for any reason pregnancy would be dangerous or ought not to occur, the Church has insisted that the husband and wife practise abstinence. And now, Nature, in offering this natural modern method of avoiding or timing pregnancy, asks only that abstinence and indulgence be timed according to certain periods in the menstrual cycle. This conforms to the laws of the Church.

In his encyclical on marriage, issued on December 31, 1930, Pope Pius XI declared: "Nor are those considered as acting against Nature who in their married life use their right in the proper manner, although on account of natural reasons of time or of certain defects, new life cannot be brought forth."

Surely this is plain. It is not "against Nature" not to have sexual union in the proper manner, and married people may have this union when they so wish.

There is a large collection of literature on this subject written from the viewpoint of the Catholic Church. In the following quotations from this literature we can hardly so much as scratch the surface.

The Very Reverend Canon Valera J. Coucke and James J. Walsh, M.D., in their book *The Sterile Period in Family Life,* bearing the Imprimatur of Patrick Cardinal Hayes, Archbishop of New York, wrote:

"As regards the purpose of marriage, we must assiduously keep in mind that the end of this institution was not that children should or even could be born in every family, but that through this institution the conservation of the species should be sufficiently provided for. As long as this preservation is not endangered, it cannot be shown that this or that couple must seek times that are propitious for pregnancy, and that they must positively intend generation. It suffices that they are perfectly faithful to the regulations of Nature. Union is permitted at the time of the agenesis (the sterile days in the menstrual cycle) just as it is allowed during pregnancy or with a woman who is sterile. . . .

Married people may deliberately choose a time at which fecundation (pregnancy) is improbable or impossible. For certain definite times will be naturally unfruitful or rarely fruitful. Married people have no obligation to make use of matrimony at the time that is propitious for fecundation and they have the privileges at any times they care to choose. Why, therefore, should people who do not wish to have children be forbidden to wait for the time which is never or rarely fruitful, provided they do not intend to disturb the order of Nature or interfere with fecundation should the latter take place contrary to their expectations? This conduct can certainly be called licit as long as the required conservation of the species is not in danger. . . . It is the plan of Nature that periods of sterility should exist."

Our Sunday Visitor, published by the Catholic Bishop of Fort Wayne, a publication having wide circulation in this country and abroad, recently devoted over a half of an issue informing its readers of this natural method of avoiding conception. This press published a small book on this subject which has enjoyed a wide distribution.

In one part of *A Handbook of Moral Theology*, by

Arthur Preuss, we read, "It is permissible to limit sexual intercourse to the period during which conception does not ordinarily take place."

Hildebrand said: "To regard wedded love as exclusively an objective means to the union of wedlock, and later in turn as a means of procreation, would be to subordinate entirely man as a human being to man as an animal . . . a thoroughly materialistic view."

What Is Marriage?—a Catechism according to the Encyclical *Casti Connubii* of Pope Pius XI, in justification of the natural method of birth-control, and in explanation of the differences between natural birth-control and contraception, and of the conditions that are to be observed, has the following passage:

"As long as the act takes place normally it remains objectively directed toward its primary end, which is generation, and since, according to the maxim that the purpose of the law is not within the matter of the law (*finis legis non cadit sub legem*), there is no obligation, while observing the law to intend the end for which it was promulgated, it follows that the act is not necessarily vitiated by deliberately choosing a certain time with the intention of avoiding conception. Of course, the couple are bound to welcome any children that might come, if, as sometimes happens, their plan fails. The conjugal intercourse, at any rate, serves the other ends of marriage.

"Besides, let us observe that there is a great difference between the practice of birth control and the restricted use of marriage of which we speak. The abuses of birth control can be practiced, constantly, they give free rein to passion, they do not demand the exercise of any moral force whatever; whereas this limited use of marriage requires, for the voluntary abstinence on certain days, a moral force the exercise of which is not without its social value.

"In itself indifferent or objectively good, this limitation which is not a violation of nature, may, according to circumstances and the intention, be praiseworthy, less desirable, or even worthy of blame."

"Accordingly, the Sacred Penitentiary, in its reply of June 16, 1880, declared that there was no reason to disturb those married people who in their use of marriage, restricted themselves to days that are physiologically sterile, and that this practice might be insinuated caute, that is with prudent discretion. With prudent discretion we say; the uncertainty of the result is enough to suggest prudence; besides, the confessor should not be a counselor of infecundity. The insinuation of this course of action may be appropriate as a means of preventing formal sins, or as offering a way out of a critical situation where the danger of incontinence makes intercourse imperative, and yet where conception would be perilous for the mother. It goes without saying that this practice normally supposes the agreement of both parties."

From our quotations it may readily be acknowledged that the Catholic Church does not object to this natural method of avoiding the consequences of a natural marital act. In other words, a married couple may have physical union whenever desired, though nothing may be done to prevent the consequences of the act. If a married couple do not wish to cohabit during the period of fertility, they do not have to do so. They have control over the time of this act. In the last analysis, if a woman wishes to avoid pregnancy, she will practise abstinence during a certain period of her menstrual cycle. But when she does have intercourse it must be natural in method, and no chemical substances may be used, nor may any mechanical devices be employed to frustrate the possible fruitfulness of the act.

For those who have read thus far and intend to practise this method, we urge the following:

1. Only women with regular menstrual cycles, or cycles which are irregular within known limits, should attempt to figure their sterile and fertile periods. Women who are irregular within uncertain wide limits, or who flow profusely and pathologically should consult a physician.

2. From the preceding chapters any woman who desires can figure out her own cycles of sterility and fecundity. However, we urge that you check your findings with your particular chart (Chap. VI.)

3. By following instructions you can use the calendar (supplied with this book) and the chart peculiar to your menstrual type, and know the exact days of any particular month on which you are fertile or sterile.

4. Menstruation ceases during the nursing period. When nursing is over, the menses usually re-appear. However, until two or three menses have occurred, no conception period can be figured. As a rule a nursing mother is sterile. A fair rule to follow is to practise abstinence when lactation ends until two or three periods have occurred and in this manner the safe and the unsafe periods in the menstrual cycle can be reckoned.

5. When pregnancy is to be avoided engage in marital union only during the sterile dates.

6. When pregnancy is desired it is best to confine

sexual union to the fertile time in the menstrual cycle. Excessive marital relations are more likely to prevent than to make it possible.

7. One must follow to the very letter the rules laid down for success in the practice of this method. No hit-or-miss method is safe; "taking a chance" invites disaster. It has been claimed that, except in the freak case, failure is the result of the woman's not having observed the laws—which must be scrupulously followed —and is not the result of the method itself.

8. This modern method calls for character, control and will-power. At the worst, it calls for abstinence for short periods of time. Will-power, abstinence, and a knowledge of the times of fertility and sterility in a woman's menstrual cycle, are all the essentials required.

In an article published in the *Journal of the American Medical Association* (Feb. 10, 1934), on "Two Important Biologic Factors in Fertility and Sterility," Emil Novak, M.D., of Johns Hopkins, and recognized here and abroad as a gynecologist of wide experience, wrote. "For those who, because of religious or other reasons, are not willing to resort to other forms of contraception, the Ogino-Knaus method is a great boon and is certainly the one that should be recommended by the physician."

From the same issue of this journal we quote part of an editorial based on Dr. Novak's contribution. The editorial is entitled "The Safe Period In Women." It reads:

"Thus there is being developed scientific evidence to warrant the possibility that this method for the prevention of conception or birth-control is sufficiently accurate to be dependable and at the same time psychologically, socially and esthetically sound. It calls for a certain amount of civilized restraint. . . . In view of the nature of the evidence now brought forward and rather well confirmed it would seem desirable that large clinics especially interested in studying the prevention of conception might concentrate their efforts temporarily on a study of this method from all different points of view that have been mentioned. *The possibilities seem more promising than promoting the sale of various mechanical devices, chemical substances and other forms of intricate manipulation which have not met any of the critical criterions that have been mentioned.*" (Italics ours.)

On September 8, 1934, an editorial in the *Journal of the American Medical Association* on natural birth-control claimed: "Enough evidence has already been established to indicate that strict observance of the method is assurance of sterility, even beyond that associated with the employment of the most of the contraceptive appliances and medicament."

"Nature is not to be governed except through obeying her." Bacon's thought covers the whole subject we have discussed.

CHAPTER VIII

THE MODERN METHOD OF BIRTH CONTROL
AFTER TWENTY YEARS

T HE FIRST EDITION of this book was published in January, 1935, and this chapter was written early in the spring of 1954. During the last two decades several hundred thousand copies of The Modern Method have been purchased. After the early advertising and book reviews the book sold itself. Physicians have recommended it to their patients, and women who found the Method reliable have told their friends and neighbors about it. It is still as dependable as any other method, whether it be a mechanical contrivance, a jelly or a chemical in a douche. Nothing is 100 per cent perfect, even surgical sterilization; pregnancy has taken place following every known means of birth control.

Since this book has been in circulation we have received hundreds of letters from women, and from a few husbands, asking for further information on some particular phase of the subject. We have also been told by some acquaintances that they have no faith in the Method. When asked the reasons for this conclusion, the usual answer is, "It seems too simple," or "they heard" of a woman who became pregnant while following the "rhythm" theory.

The Method fails in less than two per cent of the cases. However, if the failures were common occurrences, we would have received many, many letters of protest and criticism. Conservatively, upward of 300,000 women have adopted the Method, and to date we have received not more than twenty-five letters carrying complaints. On the other hand, we have received scores of letters informing us that while following the Method conception did not occur; and when another baby was desired, a reversal of the Method was crowned with success. This is not surprising, because in medical literature dealing with the problem of sterility practically every author advocates intercourse particularly during the fertile period of the menstrual cycle.

Why does the Method fail in rare instances? Some scientists affirm that some women ovulate at any time in the cycle; there are others who oppose this theory. We believe it is true, and this opinion is based on personal reports from women who have become pregnant after a single cohabitation during the sterile period. Women of this type are few and far between. Before we finish this chapter we will suggest another means of estimating ovulation time.

The greatest number of failures occur because many women do not accurately estimate or make sure of their personal cycles. They rely on a capricious memory and do not bother or take the trouble to keep accurate written records of their menstrual dates over a period of several months. Unless one has made sure of the accuracy of the shortest and longest time interval between many menstrual periods, the employment of the Method may end in failure. There is only one way to be sure on this important point and that is to keep an accurate calendar record. Do not rely on memory. It may lead you astray. Usually after a record has been tabulated for a year one will know if she menstruates "on the dot" (so many women tell their physicians they can almost predict the very hour of the day they will menstruate), or if there is a variation of one, two, three or four (or more) days. In this way any variation, even though it be slight, must be noted. This is of cardinal importance. Example: Even if one menstruates for many months every 28 days and then notes a 27- or a 29-day cycle, the cycle 27–28, 28–29 or 27–29 will be the correct one.

For the woman who has eccentric, unpredictable cycles, or the woman who may "menstruate at any time" or whose menstrual cycle varies more than four days, our advice is not to rely on the Method. The woman who follows a wrong cycle is liable to failure, as is the woman who menstruates at irregular, unpredictable times. The Method in these cases will most likely prove futile.

The question is asked, "What cycle should I follow after I have had a baby?" Usually most new mothers will have their first period from about forty to sixty days after giving birth. If menstruation does not occur after eight weeks, it is well to consult a physician. Marital

relations should not be resumed until after the first normal period following delivery. Pregnancy can and has
taken place during the period prior to the first menstruation. We have in mind the wife of a physician who
followed the Method successfully for nearly three years
after her second child. Then she became pregnant by
choice and gave birth on April 4, 1951. On February 2,
1952, she had another child. After the first post-natal
period an accurate chart or recording of the interval between periods should be kept. Meanwhile, until one is
sure of her cycle, the best she can do is to follow the cycle she followed prior to her recent or last pregnancy.
This is not an air-tight, safe method, but it is the best
one can follow. At least the chances of failure are re-
duced to a minimum. After the woman has kept a new
record for a suitable length of time, any change in her
cycle will be noted and the new cycle should be put into
practical application.

There is a popular belief among many people that
while a woman nurses a baby conception is impossible.
It is true that pregnancy is not probable during the period of nursing but it is possible. During these weeks
or months what should one do? This is a hard question
to answer. It has been suggested that the temperature
method of discovering ovulation time (should the
woman ovulate) should be followed.

The technic of this method is as follows: A special
rectal thermometer is manufactured for this purpose.
The degrees of temperature and fractions of a degree
are widely calibrated, making it possible even for the

novice to read them easily. The variations in temperature recordings are slight and fractions of a degree are important. If one is practiced at reading the standard rectal thermometer, it may be used. These special rectal thermometers can be purchased at most medical or surgical supply concerns. Should you not know of such a concern, your physician will undoubtedly know where to refer you.

You can either get a printed temperature chart (at the same concern) or make one yourself. Draw small squares on a large sheet of paper. Make a heavy line for each degree of temperature, and allow five perpendicular squares for temperatures of a fifth of a degree between the heavy lines. Each horizontal square represents one day. Number them at the top.

Every morning on awakening in bed insert the thermometer in the rectum. Keep it there for five minutes. Then read the temperature. Mark it with a dot in the proper square on the chart. Connect the dots from day to day with a straight line. This line will not be even. The result will look not unlike the temperature chart of a convalescing patient in a hospital. At first the recording will be represented by a fluctuating low curve. The temperature may and usually is slightly subnormal. About the time of ovulation the curve drops and then rises to a higher level which is maintained until the next menstruation. There is a difference of opinion as to whether ovulation occurs at the time of the drop or at the time of the rise in temperature. For practical purposes it is generally believed that the egg leaves the ovary at this time. Often, with a little practice, one becomes quite expert in determining the time of ovulation by this basal temperature method. Unfortunately, some women run an unusual temperature curve, and only one with a wide knowledge and experience in this work can be depended on to reach the correct answers. If you cannot make head or tail of these temperature recordings, our advice is to seek the assistance of a physician conversant with such matters. (Do not write to the author.)

The rectal temperature method may be of inestimable help to women who cannot employ the Method due to abnormal or wide variations in menstrual cycles, during lactation (the period in which the baby is nursed), or women who wish to conceive and for some reason fail to ovulate or cannot figure the time in the cycle when ovulation occurs.

Now that this subject has been brought up-to-date and you have learned about its use in overcoming sterility, how to apply the Method and when not to follow it, why in a minimum of instances it may fail, how to overcome such failures and how to determine ovulation periods when nursing a baby, disappointment should not be your lot if you follow these rules.

> [*Short inquiries will be answered provided they are accompanied by a stamped, self-addressed envelope.*]

CHAPTER IX

MENSTRUAL CALENDARS

THE FOLLOWING menstrual calendars are offered for a specific reason. It is not advisable to leave the actual dates of menstruation to one's memory. Many women change in type from time to time. Inasmuch as the absolute length of the menstrual cycle is important in determining the periods of fertility and sterility, it is urged that a notation is made on the calendars of the date of the beginning of each menstruation.

1955

JANUARY

SUN.	MON.	TUES.	WED.	THUR.	FRI.	SAT.
						1
2	3	4	5	6	7	8
9	10	11	12	13	14	15
16	17	18	19	20	21	22
23	24	25	26	27	28	29
30	31					

FEBRUARY

SUN.	MON.	TUES.	WED.	THUR.	FRI.	SAT.
		1	2	3	4	5
6	7	8	9	10	11	12
13	14	15	16	17	18	19
20	21	22	23	24	25	26
27	28					

MARCH

SUN.	MON.	TUES.	WED.	THUR.	FRI.	SAT.
		1	2	3	4	5
6	7	8	9	10	11	12
13	14	15	16	17	18	19
20	21	22	23	24	25	26
27	28	29	30	31		

APRIL

SUN.	MON.	TUES.	WED.	THUR.	FRI.	SAT.
					1	2
3	4	5	6	7	8	9
10	11	12	13	14	15	16
17	18	19	20	21	22	23
24	25	26	27	28	29	30

MAY

SUN.	MON.	TUES.	WED.	THUR.	FRI.	SAT.
1	2	3	4	5	6	7
8	9	10	11	12	13	14
15	16	17	18	19	20	21
22	23	24	25	26	27	28
29	30	31				

JUNE

SUN.	MON.	TUES.	WED.	THUR.	FRI.	SAT.
			1	2	3	4
5	6	7	8	9	10	11
12	13	14	15	16	17	18
19	20	21	22	23	24	25
26	27	28	29	30		

JULY

SUN.	MON.	TUES.	WED.	THUR.	FRI.	SAT.
					1	2
3	4	5	6	7	8	9
10	11	12	13	14	15	16
17	18	19	20	21	22	23
24	25	26	27	28	29	30
31						

AUGUST

SUN.	MON.	TUES.	WED.	THUR.	FRI.	SAT.
	1	2	3	4	5	6
7	8	9	10	11	12	13
14	15	16	17	18	19	20
21	22	23	24	25	26	27
28	29	30	31			

SEPTEMBER

SUN.	MON.	TUES.	WED.	THUR.	FRI.	SAT.
				1	2	3
4	5	6	7	8	9	10
11	12	13	14	15	16	17
18	19	20	21	22	23	24
25	26	27	28	29	30	

OCTOBER

SUN.	MON.	TUES.	WED.	THUR.	FRI.	SAT.
						1
2	3	4	5	6	7	8
9	10	11	12	13	14	15
16	17	18	19	20	21	22
23	24	25	26	27	28	29
30	31					

NOVEMBER

SUN.	MON.	TUES.	WED.	THUR.	FRI.	SAT.
		1	2	3	4	5
6	7	8	9	10	11	12
13	14	15	16	17	18	19
20	21	22	23	24	25	26
27	28	29	30			

DECEMBER

SUN.	MON.	TUES.	WED.	THUR.	FRI.	SAT.
				1	2	3
4	5	6	7	8	9	10
11	12	13	14	15	16	17
18	19	20	21	22	23	24
25	26	27	28	29	30	31

1956

JANUARY

SUN.	MON.	TUES.	WED.	THUR.	FRI.	SAT.
1	2	3	4	5	6	7
8	9	10	11	12	13	14
15	16	17	18	19	20	21
22	23	24	25	26	27	28
29	30	31				

FEBRUARY

SUN.	MON.	TUES.	WED.	THUR.	FRI.	SAT.
			1	2	3	4
5	6	7	8	9	10	11
12	13	14	15	16	17	18
19	20	21	22	23	24	25
26	27	28	29			

MARCH

SUN.	MON.	TUES.	WED.	THUR.	FRI.	SAT.
				1	2	3
4	5	6	7	8	9	10
11	12	13	14	15	16	17
18	19	20	21	22	23	24
25	26	27	28	29	30	31

APRIL

SUN.	MON.	TUES.	WED.	THUR.	FRI.	SAT.
1	2	3	4	5	6	7
8	9	10	11	12	13	14
15	16	17	18	19	20	21
22	23	24	25	26	27	28
29	30					

MAY

SUN.	MON.	TUES.	WED.	THUR.	FRI.	SAT.
		1	2	3	4	5
6	7	8	9	10	11	12
13	14	15	16	17	18	19
20	21	22	23	24	25	26
27	28	29	30	31		

JUNE

SUN.	MON.	TUES.	WED.	THUR.	FRI.	SAT.
					1	2
3	4	5	6	7	8	9
10	11	12	13	14	15	16
17	18	19	20	21	22	23
24	25	26	27	28	29	30

JULY

SUN.	MON.	TUES.	WED.	THUR.	FRI.	SAT.
1	2	3	4	5	6	7
8	9	10	11	12	13	14
15	16	17	18	19	20	21
22	23	24	25	26	27	28
29	30	31				

AUGUST

SUN.	MON.	TUES.	WED.	THUR.	FRI.	SAT.
			1	2	3	4
5	6	7	8	9	10	11
12	13	14	15	16	17	18
19	20	21	22	23	24	25
26	27	28	29	30	31	

SEPTEMBER

SUN.	MON.	TUES.	WED.	THUR.	FRI.	SAT.
						1
2	3	4	5	6	7	8
9	10	11	12	13	14	15
16	17	18	19	20	21	22
23	24	25	26	27	28	29
30						

OCTOBER

SUN.	MON.	TUES.	WED.	THUR.	FRI.	SAT.
	1	2	3	4	5	6
7	8	9	10	11	12	13
14	15	16	17	18	19	20
21	22	23	24	25	26	27
28	29	30	31			

NOVEMBER

SUN.	MON.	TUES.	WED.	THUR.	FRI.	SAT.
				1	2	3
4	5	6	7	8	9	10
11	12	13	14	15	16	17
18	19	20	21	22	23	24
25	26	27	28	29	30	

DECEMBER

SUN.	MON.	TUES.	WED.	THUR.	FRI.	SAT.
						1
2	3	4	5	6	7	8
9	10	11	12	13	14	15
16	17	18	19	20	21	22
23	24	(25)	26	27	28	29
30	31					

1957

JANUARY

SUN.	MON.	TUES.	WED.	THUR.	FRI.	SAT.
		1	2	3	4	5
6	7	8	9	10	11	12
13	14	15	16	17	18	19
20	21	22	23	24	25	26
27	28	29	30	31		

FEBRUARY

SUN.	MON.	TUES.	WED.	THUR.	FRI.	SAT.
					1	2
3	4	5	6	7	8	9
10	11	12	13	14	15	16
17	18	19	20	21	22	23
24	25	26	27	28		

MARCH

SUN.	MON.	TUES.	WED.	THUR.	FRI.	SAT.
					1	2
3	4	5	6	7	8	9
10	11	12	13	14	15	16
17	18	19	20	21	22	(23)
24	25	26	27	28	29	30
31						

APRIL

SUN.	MON.	TUES.	WED.	THUR.	FRI.	SAT.
	1	2	3	4	5	6
7	8	9	10	11	12	13
14	15	16	17	18	(19)	20
21	22	23	24	25	26	27
28	29	30				

MAY

SUN.	MON.	TUES.	WED.	THUR.	FRI.	SAT.
			1	2	3	4
5	6	7	8	9	10	11
12	13	14	(15)	16	17	(18)
19	20	21	22	23	24	25
26	27	28	29	30	31	

JUNE

SUN.	MON.	TUES.	WED.	THUR.	FRI.	SAT.
						1
2	3	4	5	6	7	8
9	10	11	12	13	14	15
16	17	18	19	20	21	22
23	(24)	25	26	27	28	29
30						

JULY

SUN.	MON.	TUES.	WED.	THUR.	FRI.	SAT.
	1	2	3	4	5	6
7	8	9	10	11	12	13
14	15	16	17	18	19	20
21	22	23	24	25	26	27
28	29	30	31			

AUGUST

SUN.	MON.	TUES.	WED.	THUR.	FRI.	SAT.
				1	2	3
4	5	6	7	8	9	10
11	12	13	14	15	16	17
18	19	20	21	22	23	24
25	26	27	28	29	30	31

SEPTEMBER

SUN.	MON.	TUES.	WED.	THUR.	FRI.	SAT.
1	2	3	4	5	6	7
8	9	10	11	12	13	14
15	16	17	18	19	20	21
22	23	24	25	26	27	28
29	30					

OCTOBER

SUN.	MON.	TUES.	WED.	THUR.	FRI.	SAT.
		1	2	3	4	5
6	7	8	9	10	11	12
13	14	15	16	17	18	19
20	21	22	23	24	25	26
27	28	29	30	31		

NOVEMBER

SUN.	MON.	TUES.	WED.	THUR.	FRI.	SAT.
					1	2
3	4	5	6	7	8	9
10	11	12	13	14	15	16
17	18	19	20	21	22	23
24	25	26	27	28	29	30

DECEMBER

SUN.	MON.	TUES.	WED.	THUR.	FRI.	SAT.
1	2	3	4	5	6	7
8	9	10	11	12	13	14
15	16	17	18	19	20	21
22	23	24	25	26	27	28
29	30	31				

1958

JANUARY

SUN.	MON.	TUES.	WED.	THUR.	FRI.	SAT.
			1	2	3	4
5	6	7	8	9	10	11
12	13	14	15	16	17	18
19	20	21	22	23	24	25
26	27	28	29	30	31	

FEBRUARY

SUN.	MON.	TUES.	WED.	THUR.	FRI.	SAT.
						1
2	3	4	5	6	7	8
9	10	11	12	13	14	15
16	17	18	19	20	21	22
23	24	25	26	27	28	

MARCH

SUN.	MON.	TUES.	WED.	THUR.	FRI.	SAT.
						1
2	3	4	5	6	7	8
9	10	11	12	13	14	15
16	17	18	19	20	21	22
23	24	25	26	27	28	29
30	31					

APRIL

SUN.	MON.	TUES.	WED.	THUR.	FRI.	SAT.
		1	2	3	4	5
6	7	8	9	10	11	12
13	14	15	16	17	18	19
20	21	22	23	24	25	26
27	28	29	30			

MAY

SUN.	MON.	TUES.	WED.	THUR.	FRI.	SAT.
				1	2	3
4	5	6	7	8	9	10
11	12	13	14	15	16	17
18	19	20	21	22	23	24
25	26	27	28	29	30	31

JUNE

SUN.	MON.	TUES.	WED.	THUR.	FRI.	SAT.
1	2	3	4	5	6	7
8	9	10	11	12	13	14
15	16	17	18	19	20	21
22	23	24	25	26	27	28
29	30					

JULY

SUN.	MON.	TUES.	WED.	THUR.	FRI.	SAT.
		1	2	3	4	5
6	7	8	9	10	11	12
13	14	15	16	17	18	19
20	21	22	23	24	25	26
27	28	29	30	31		

AUGUST

SUN.	MON.	TUES.	WED.	THUR.	FRI.	SAT.
					1	2
3	4	5	6	7	8	9
10	11	12	13	14	15	16
17	18	19	20	21	22	23
24	25	26	27	28	29	30
31						

SEPTEMBER

SUN.	MON.	TUES.	WED.	THUR.	FRI.	SAT.
	1	2	3	4	5	6
7	8	9	10	11	12	13
14	15	16	17	18	19	20
21	22	23	24	25	26	27
28	29	30				

OCTOBER

SUN.	MON.	TUES.	WED.	THUR.	FRI.	SAT.
			1	2	3	4
5	6	7	8	9	10	11
12	13	14	15	16	17	18
19	20	21	22	23	24	25
26	27	28	29	30	31	

NOVEMBER

SUN.	MON.	TUES.	WED.	THUR.	FRI.	SAT.
						1
2	3	4	5	6	7	8
9	10	11	12	13	14	15
16	17	18	19	20	21	22
23	24	25	26	27	28	29
30						

DECEMBER

SUN.	MON.	TUES.	WED.	THUR.	FRI.	SAT.
	1	2	3	4	5	6
7	8	9	10	11	12	13
14	15	16	17	18	19	20
21	22	23	24	25	26	27
28	29	30	31			

1959

JANUARY

SUN.	MON.	TUES.	WED.	THUR.	FRI.	SAT.
				1	2	3
4	5	6	7	8	9	10
11	12	13	14	15	16	17
18	19	20	21	22	23	24
25	26	27	28	29	30	31

FEBRUARY

SUN.	MON.	TUES.	WED.	THUR.	FRI.	SAT.
1	2	3	4	5	6	7
8	9	10	11	12	13	14
15	16	17	18	19	20	21
22	23	24	25	26	27	28

MARCH

SUN.	MON.	TUES.	WED.	THUR.	FRI.	SAT.
1	2	3	4	5	6	7
8	9	10	11	12	13	14
15	16	17	18	19	20	21
22	23	24	25	26	27	28
29	30	31				

APRIL

SUN.	MON.	TUES.	WED.	THUR.	FRI.	SAT.
			1	2	3	4
5	6	7	8	9	10	11
12	13	14	15	16	17	18
19	20	21	22	23	24	25
26	27	28	29	30		

MAY

SUN.	MON.	TUES.	WED.	THUR.	FRI.	SAT.
					1	2
3	4	5	6	7	8	9
10	11	12	13	14	15	16
17	18	19	20	21	22	23
24	25	26	27	28	29	30
31						

JUNE

SUN.	MON.	TUES.	WED.	THUR.	FRI.	SAT.
	1	2	3	4	5	6
7	8	9	10	11	12	13
14	15	16	17	18	19	20
21	22	23	24	25	26	27
28	29	30				

JULY

SUN.	MON.	TUES.	WED.	THUR.	FRI.	SAT.
			1	2	3	4
5	6	7	8	9	10	11
12	13	14	15	16	17	18
19	20	21	22	23	24	25
26	27	28	29	30	31	

AUGUST

SUN.	MON.	TUES.	WED.	THUR.	FRI.	SAT.
						1
2	3	4	5	6	7	8
9	10	11	12	13	14	15
16	17	18	19	20	21	22
23	24	25	26	27	28	29
30	31					

SEPTEMBER

SUN.	MON.	TUES.	WED.	THUR.	FRI.	SAT.
		1	2	3	4	5
6	7	8	9	10	11	12
13	14	15	16	17	18	19
20	21	22	23	24	25	26
27	28	29	30			

OCTOBER

SUN.	MON.	TUES.	WED.	THUR.	FRI.	SAT.
				1	2	3
4	5	6	7	8	9	10
11	12	13	14	15	16	17
18	19	20	21	22	23	24
25	26	27	28	29	30	31

NOVEMBER

SUN.	MON.	TUES.	WED.	THUR.	FRI.	SAT.
1	2	3	4	5	6	7
8	9	10	11	12	13	14
15	16	17	18	19	20	21
22	23	24	25	26	27	28
29	30					

DECEMBER

SUN.	MON.	TUES.	WED.	THUR.	FRI.	SAT.
		1	2	3	4	5
6	7	8	9	10	11	12
13	14	15	16	17	18	19
20	21	22	23	24	25	26
27	28	29	30	31		